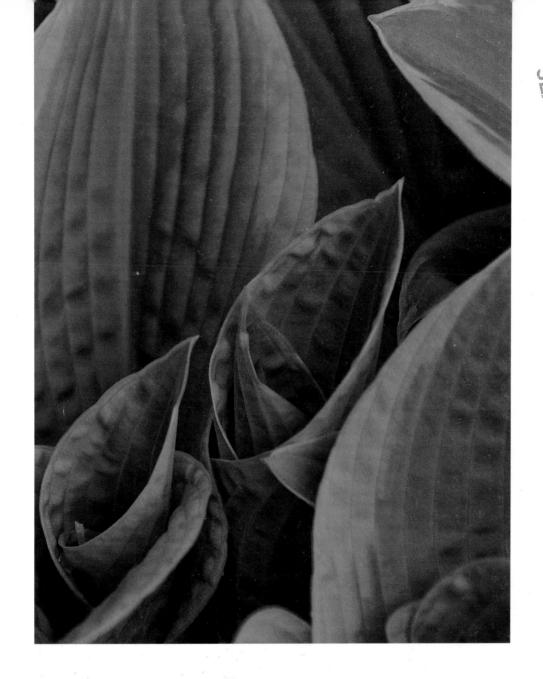

 OPEN SPACES
SACRED PLACES

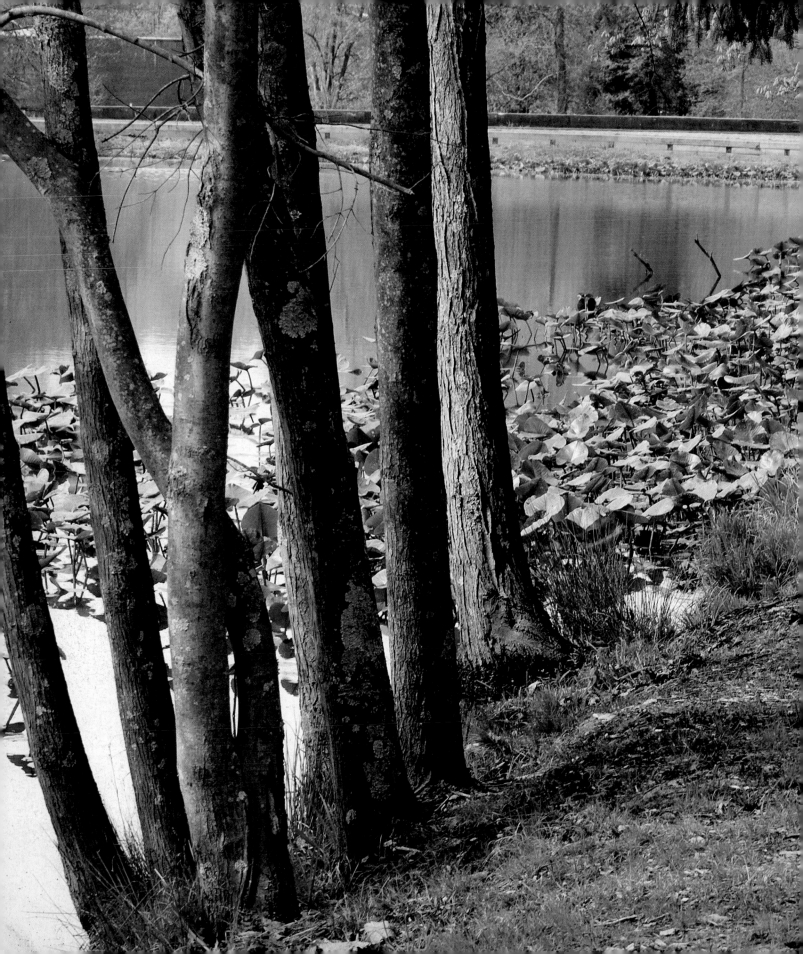

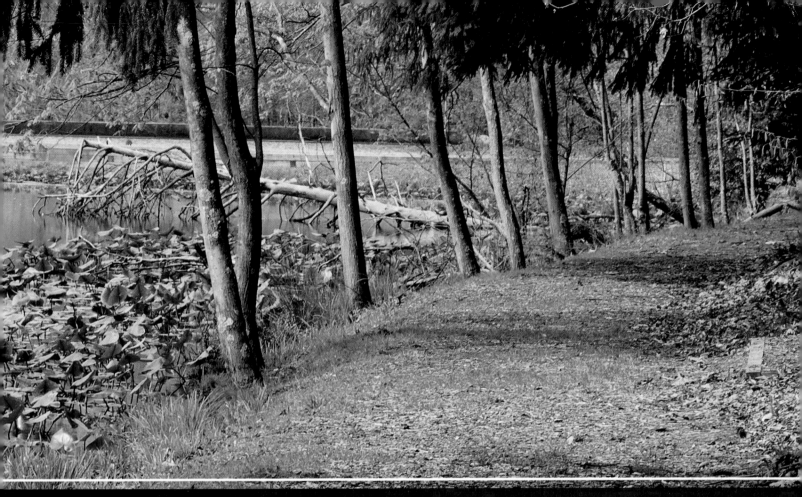

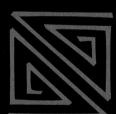 # OPEN SPACES
SACRED PLACES^{SM}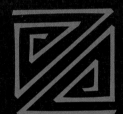

STORIES OF HOW NATURE HEALS AND UNIFIES

TOM STONER AND CAROLYN RAPP

WITH A FOREWORD BY G. MARTIN MOELLER JR.

All proceeds from the sale of this book will go to creating open spaces sacred places.

The mission of the TKF Foundation is to provide the opportunity
for a deeper human experience by supporting the creation of public
greenspaces that offer a temporary place of sanctuary, encourage
reflection, provide solace, and engender peace.

Published by TKF Foundation
410 Severn Avenue, Suite 216
Annapolis, MD 21403
www.tkffdn.org
www.openspacessacredplaces.org

Distributed by Chelsea Green Publishing
P.O. Box 428
85 N. Main Street, Suite 120
White River Junction, VT 05001
www.chelseagreen.com

Designed by Alex Castro, Castro/Arts, Baltimore

Printed by R. R. Donnelley & Sons Company
on 10% PCW-FSC Certified paper

ISBN: 978-0-9815656-0-6

Publisher's Cataloging-In-Publication Data
(Prepared by The Donohue Group, Inc.)

Stoner, Tom (Tom H.)
  Open spaces sacred places℠: stories of how nature heals and unifies /
by Tom Stoner and Carolyn Rapp ; with a foreword by G. Martin Moeller Jr.

  p. : ill. ; cm.

  ISBN: 978-0-9815656-0-6

1. Sanctuary gardens. 2. Nature, Healing power of. 3. Open spaces.
I. Rapp, Carolyn Freas. II. Moeller, Gerard Martin. III. Title.

SB454.3.S25 S76 2008
712   2008904150

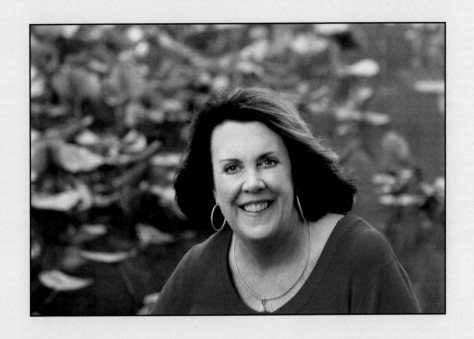

THIS BOOK IS DEDICATED TO

MARY F. WYATT

OUR FOUNDING FIRESOUL

WHO NURTURED THESE STORIES AND THESE
OPEN SPACES SACRED PLACES
INTO CREATION.

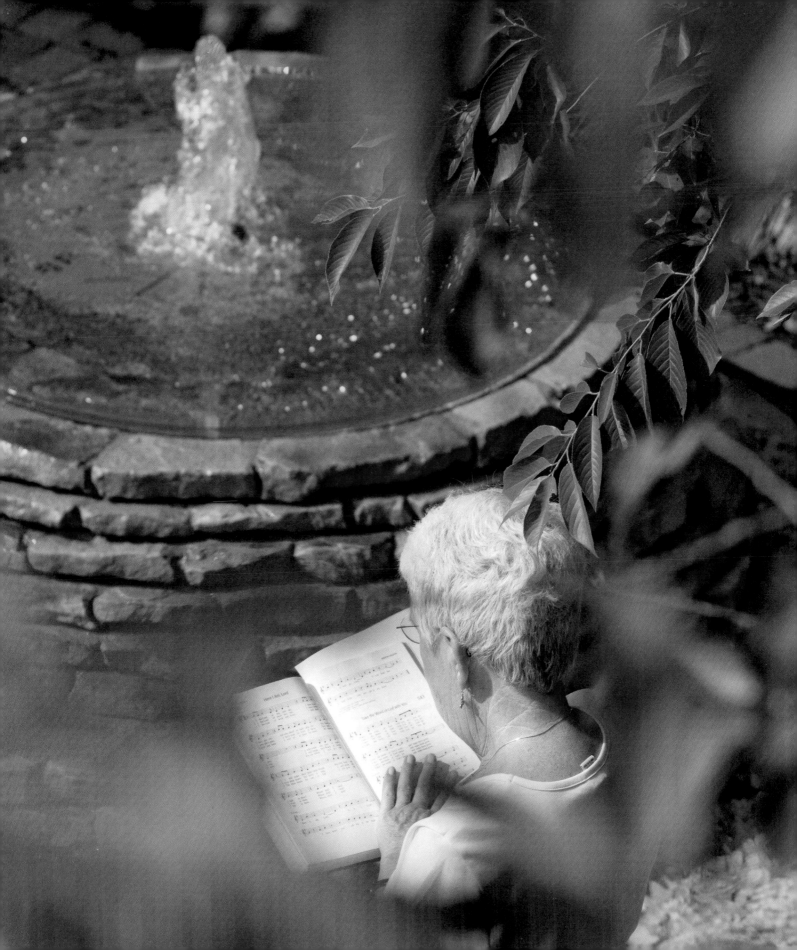

CONTENTS

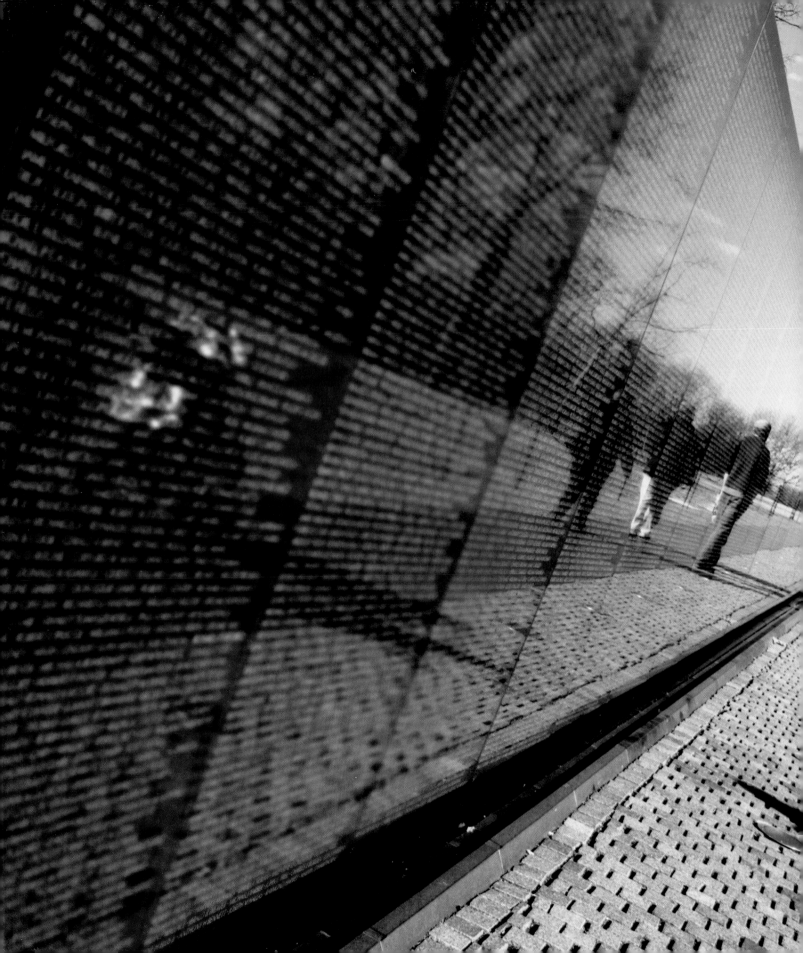

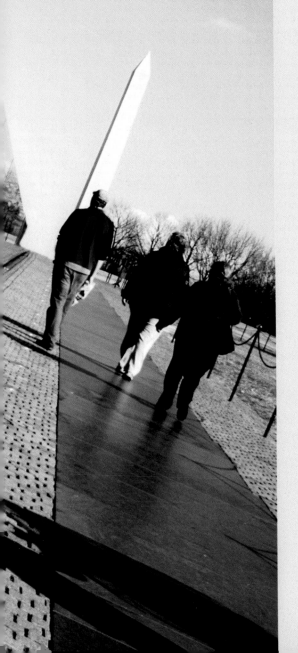

Foreword

G. Martin Moeller Jr.

Senior Vice President and Curator, National Building Museum

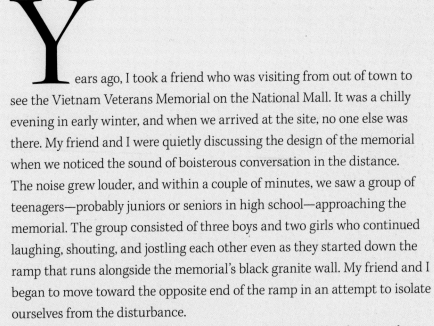

Years ago, I took a friend who was visiting from out of town to see the Vietnam Veterans Memorial on the National Mall. It was a chilly evening in early winter, and when we arrived at the site, no one else was there. My friend and I were quietly discussing the design of the memorial when we noticed the sound of boisterous conversation in the distance. The noise grew louder, and within a couple of minutes, we saw a group of teenagers—probably juniors or seniors in high school—approaching the memorial. The group consisted of three boys and two girls who continued laughing, shouting, and jostling each other even as they started down the ramp that runs alongside the memorial's black granite wall. My friend and I began to move toward the opposite end of the ramp in an attempt to isolate ourselves from the disturbance.

Before long, however, the commotion subsided, and by the time the teenagers reached the apex of the chevron-shaped wall, they were completely silent. Several of them gradually split off from the group—two of the girls walking slowly while lightly touching the wall, one boy going off to sit by himself on the grass nearby. Meanwhile, one of the boys who remained at the apex stretched out both of his arms and placed his palms flat against the two faces of the wall and held them there for perhaps a full minute. A few moments later, the group gathered again at the center and began conversing so quietly that neither my friend nor I could hear what they were saying. Eventually, they walked slowly up the ramp and left the site. As they did so, we could hear the volume of their voices increase and could once again make out some of their words, but the conversation remained far more sedate in tone and substance than it had been when they arrived.

My friend and I were both struck by the impact of the memorial on these young people. The teenagers, who had probably faced little tragedy in their lives and were likely far more concerned with their own social and hormonal challenges than with the meaning of a past geopolitical conflict, were clearly moved by their visit. They had carefully studied the texture of the wall and had turned their heads in an effort to comprehend its scale—one of them had even gestured to his friends when he discovered the reflections of the nearby Washington Monument and Lincoln Memorial in the polished granite surface.

No one told these exuberant teenagers to behave respectfully at this somber site—no one had to. That is because the Vietnam Veterans Memorial commands reverence and invites contemplation by virtue of its setting, its subject matter, and above all, its design. It is, in short, a sacred place.

After Tom Stoner invited me to write the foreword to this book, I confessed to him that I was uncomfortable with the word *sacred*. He smiled and nodded, acknowledging that it is indeed a problematic term, thanks to its religious connotations, and can mean drastically different things to different people. And yet no other word seems as apt to describe the ineffable qualities that make places like the Vietnam Veterans Memorial and the gardens and courtyards featured in this book so special. Sacred places are those that have a power—subtle though it may be—to inspire fruitful introspection, to promote emotional and even physical well-being, or simply to provide a respite from the rigors of daily life.

I was intrigued by Tom's account of the small park in London that he and his wife, Kitty, discovered by accident, and which ultimately inspired their initiative to support the creation of new sacred places. His description reminded me of dozens of similarly modest but beautiful urban spaces I had encountered in my own travels, particularly in Europe and Latin America. Although I am strongly attracted to big, bustling, even chaotic cities, some of my fondest memories involve quiet little urban oases that I happened upon by chance—a secret garden in the French Quarter in New Orleans; an inexplicably undeveloped triangle of grass in New York's Greenwich Village; a tiny, moonlit piazza in Venice where I saw a young couple dressed in evening clothes dancing to a romantic song on the radio.

Tom went on to explain that he and Kitty had gone back to that London park several times to assess what made it so successful as an urban space.

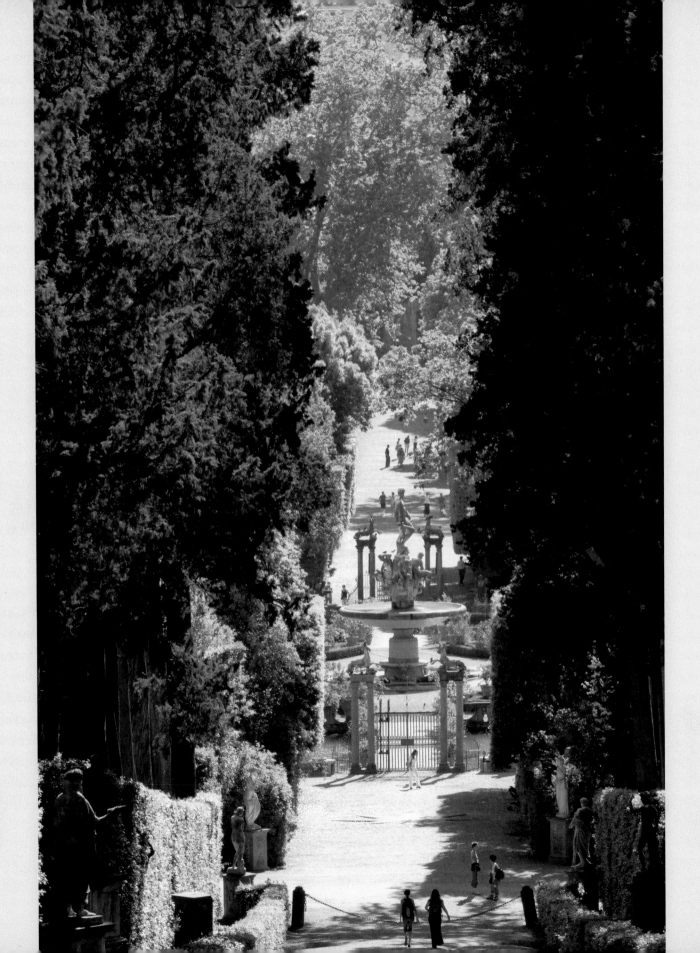

Perhaps most obvious was that it offered a comforting enclosure, complemented by a well-defined portal that marked the transition from the hectic city to the quiet enclave. Informal paths encouraged movement throughout the space, while benches provided welcome spots for visitors to rest or think. Particularly intriguing were the plaques placed on the backs of the benches, containing text that revealed aspects of the park's social history, which otherwise might have remained completely invisible to the casual modern-day visitor.

Several of the design elements that the Stoners identified in the park resonate with ideas put forth by influential urban designers and theoreticians over the past century and a quarter—including Camillo Sitte, an Austrian architect who in 1889 wrote a book later published in English as *City Planning According to Artistic Principles*; Jane Jacobs, author of the 1961 classic *The Death and Life of Great American Cities*; and William H. Whyte, whose *The Social Life of Small Urban Spaces* was published in 1980. Sitte argued that urban spaces should be conceived as outdoor rooms, with a strong sense of enclosure and carefully planned proportions. Although focused on large-scale civic plazas, Sitte's book ultimately established a broad theoretical foundation for an approach to urban design in which purely pragmatic considerations would not trump aesthetic ones. Complementing Sitte's artistic arguments, Jacobs' and Whyte's books illuminated the sociological and psychological aspects of urban spaces, and thereby reaffirmed the value of vibrant streetscapes and neighborhoods at a time when American cities, in particular, were widely seen as moribund.

To architects, landscape architects, urban planners, and others who pay close attention to the intersections between the natural and human-made environments, the elements that Tom and Kitty identified in that London park should come as no surprise. They are the building blocks of countless successful open spaces all over the world—some of them thriving commercial or civic nodes; others tranquil, pastoral landscapes. And yet such welcoming public spaces are all too rare in the present day, particularly in the United States, where relentless suburban sprawl has sapped many cities of their vitality while gobbling up farmland and forests. Despite broad agreement about the value of open space and many excellent examples of historic and modern public places around the world, efforts to create well-designed outdoor spaces—especially small ones—are often thwarted by profound economic, political, technological, and social pressures.

In that context, the TKF Foundation's campaign to support the creation of modestly sized, human-friendly open spaces may seem quixotic.

But as Winifred Gallagher notes in her book *The Power of Place: How Our Surroundings Shape Our Thoughts, Emotions, and Actions*, originally published in 1993, the environmental movement has placed steadily increasing emphasis on the value of small gestures on the part of many individuals in protecting the natural world—a trend that has only accelerated since *sustainability* and *going green* have become buzz terms over the past few years. Gallagher points out that people tend to focus a great deal of attention on their homes, making sure that they are clean and attractive, for instance. She concludes by saying, "Once we realize that just about anything that is true of our relationship with our homes is true concerning our neighborhoods, regions, and nations, then thinking locally will mean acting globally, and that means saving the world."

The people who created the spaces featured in this book may not have set out to save the world, but they are certainly working hard to make parts of it as pleasant, meaningful, and healthful as possible—and more power to them.

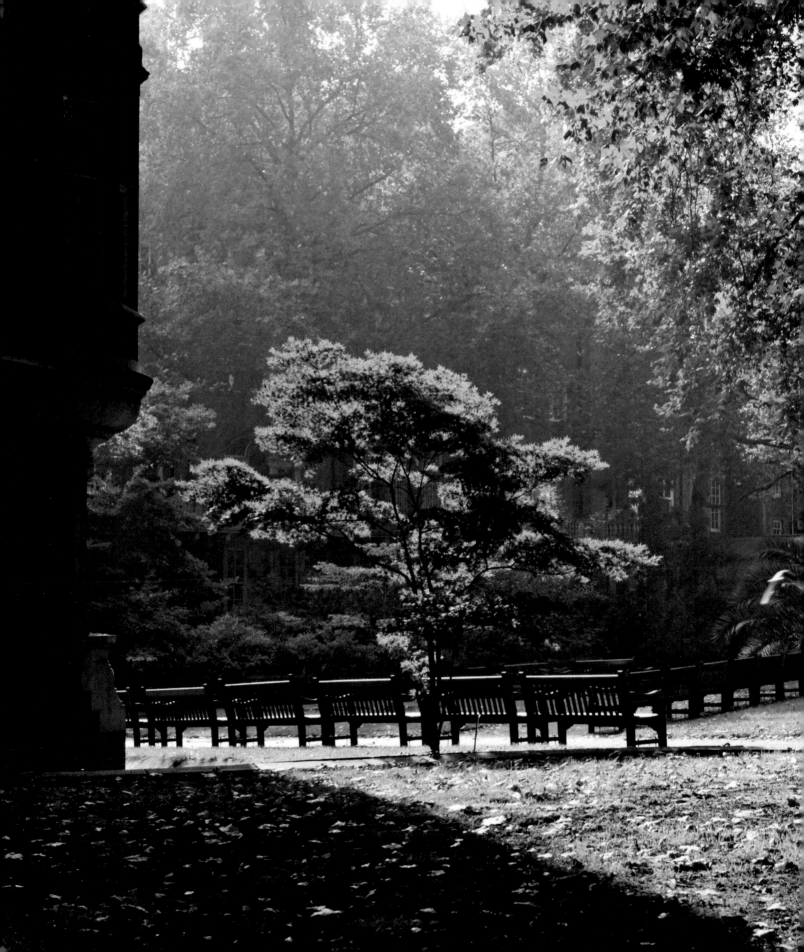

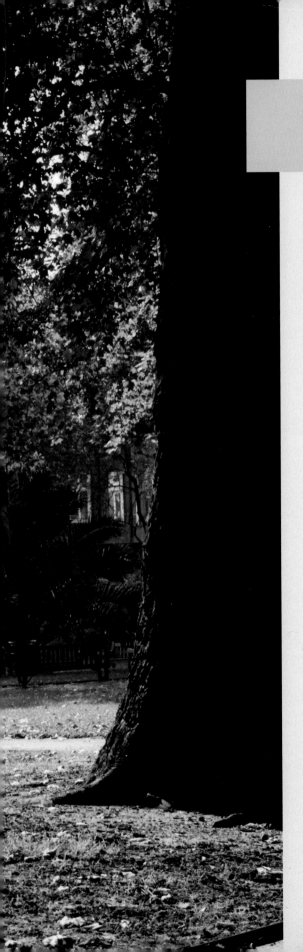

Portal to Discovery

"Climb the mountains and get their good tidings. Nature's peace will flow into you as sunshine flows into trees. The winds will blow their own freshness into you, and the storms their energy, while cares will drop away from you like the leaves of autumn."

—John Muir

Inspiration comes in amazing ways. For my wife, Kitty, and me, it was a chance visit to a London park more than a decade ago.

After a long journey across the Atlantic, Kitty and I arrived in London, too early in the day for our hotel room to be ready. In an effort to pass time and to revive ourselves after hours strapped in an airplane, we happened upon an enclosed garden in the center of the city. It was nestled amidst a ring of four-story buildings; to enter, we had to pass through a dark-red brick arch. We instantly felt as though we had left the city behind and had entered a place of serenity.

Inside, towering plane trees canopied little paths that meandered throughout the garden. Weathered benches were sprinkled along the paths, and we soon discovered that each bench had a plaque affixed to the back. The writing on the plaques offered a narrative of the generations of people who had sat there together. They not only memorialized the community that existed there over the years; they also made us realize that this was considered a place of safety and stillness, especially in times of great stress and destruction. This quiet park called Mount Street Gardens had survived

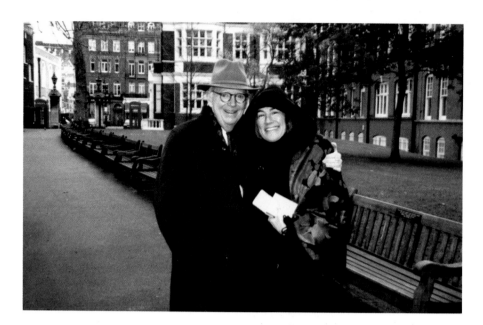

the Blitz of London during World War II and the times of terrorism that followed. The writing on the plaques revealed how the healing power of nature had given the residents a few moments of peace in a city besieged.

We had an epiphany. We realized then and there that the space was much more than just a public garden. That insight was the culmination of something that both of us had experienced in our lives, but had not quite named: the idea that certain spaces can transform you, that certain spaces are sacred.

I realize now that I had been building toward this revelation for much of my life. When I was seventeen, my father died, and I struggled to make sense of the world and my place in it. I soon found myself pressing into the Boundary Waters Canoe Area Wilderness between the United States and Canada, an enormous international ecosystem filled with lakes and streams, a place that does not permit motorboats. Leaving all technology behind, with only a canoe, paddle, backpack, and compass, I headed toward the center of the wilderness.

Perhaps it was the human effort it took to reach that center that made this place so special for me. Every rhythmic stroke of the paddle against the water took me farther into the vast unknown. It removed me from the rapid changes that were happening back home and gave me the emotional breathing room I needed to search for life's meaning and my own personal path. Nature surrounded me and helped me feel safe and whole.

Ironically, it was technology that would lead me into adulthood. I began working in the fast-paced media world, which took me in the absolute opposite direction from nature. I built a career in mass communications and watched as new information technology, from the Internet to the iPod, began to trans-

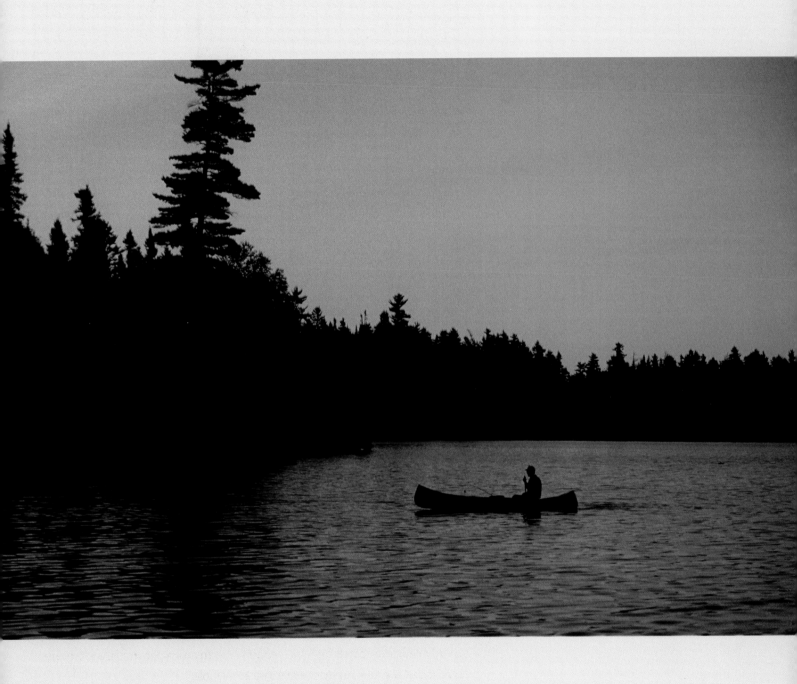

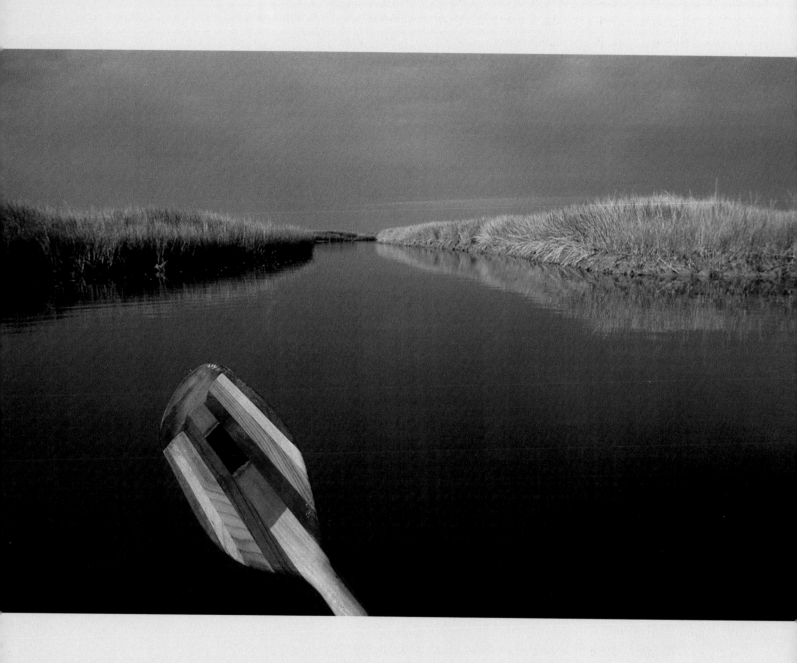

form our lives. The paradox, of course, is that the more technology claims to build community—the more technology "betters" our lives—the more isolated we all truly become. I began to realize that there is a great social cost to all of us immersed in this information and media revolution. The average American spends hours a day plugged into television, radio, the Internet. Stress, depression, and anxiety are at all-time highs. This evolution of connectivity has, in truth, disconnected us—not only from our neighbors, but also from ourselves.

I experienced this in my own life, for it was nearly always in fast-forward. Throughout my career, I often felt like a *human doing*. But I often yearned for that special place in nature where I could be a *human being* again. The memory of the Boundary Waters never left me.

I found a kindred spirit in my wife, Kitty. She grew up in a dynamic and vibrant family of five. They spent summers at a compound called Shawondasee, named by Native Americans. It was nestled in the bluffs overlooking the mighty Mississippi River. When her life's interest and training became focused on helping bring wellness to those who suffer, it impelled her to introduce the power of nature into the process of healing.

For both of us, being around water, mountains, and meadows became an essential part of our lives. Whenever possible, we biked, hiked, paddled, and sailed. We brought this love and appreciation of nature with us as we moved from the Midwest to the eastern seaboard. We decided to live as close to nature as possible and chose land near the waters of the Chesapeake Bay in Maryland. As time passed and success came, we began to ask ourselves how we could share with others the healing power of the natural world that had so blessed us throughout our lives. We began to think of this search as a pilgrimage.

Standing in Mount Street Gardens in London, Kitty and I felt we had found an answer. We knew we were in a sacred space. The writing on the benches told us so. It was clear that the writers had taken the opportunity to reflect on what was happening in their world and that they had wanted to share their reflections. We felt an urgent call to help foster places like this one. For the first time in human history, more than half of the world's population lives in an urban setting. By 2030, those numbers could tip to more than 60 percent. The world is rapidly changing, and not all of us have the opportunity to take to the Boundary Waters in times of emotional crises.

Kitty and I suddenly, quite clearly, understood the vital and varied role that a sacred space can play in our hectic lives. Such a place can serve to do something as simple as salve two weary travelers or something as complex as spark a spiritual awakening. Whatever the result, the space itself has facilitated that end.

So what makes an environment capable of that kind of transformation? At the heart of it is a thoughtful plan wedded in the belief that the design of a space has the capacity to empower the people within its confines. London writer Alain de Botton put it this way in his book *The Architecture of Happiness:* "Belief in the significance of architecture is premised on the notion that we are, for better or for worse, different people in different places—and on the conviction that it is architecture's task to render vivid to us who we might ideally be."

For the rest of our stay and on the way back home to America, we tried to integrate what we had experienced in that park into a plan for action. We analyzed the physical components that helped foster such a powerful moment, one that echoed the feelings of being in nature. We began to conceive of the design elements that went into making that park a sacred space. First, there was the portal that we physically walked through to enter the garden. Then there was the surround, or enclosure, that helped the park feel safe and inviting. There were the paths that encouraged exploration and introspection. There were the destination points, the benches, which offered a place to rest, reflect, and connect with the many visitors who had been there before us. And finally, and most importantly, there was the openness—the space was open to anyone who cared to walk its verdant paths.

We wanted to help create these open spaces and sacred places in our own community, and so the TKF Foundation was born. Back home, we invited a great number of environmentalists, sociologists, architects, people of faith, and community activists from all across America to help write our mission statement. They were the kindred spirits who helped us articulate the TKF mission: "to provide the opportunity for a deeper human experience by supporting the creation of public greenspaces that offer a temporary place of sanctuary, encourage reflection, provide solace, and engender peace."

We encouraged these same leaders and many more to propose implementation of this mission. We did not tell them where these spaces needed to exist; we simply charged them with seeking sites that could be transformed. We did limit our geography. Kitty and I decided early on to focus our energies within the Mid-Atlantic area. In this way, the various participants would have the ability to connect and learn from one another. Kitty and I visualized this effort to be a Petri dish of experimentation, and that is what it has become.

We have been awed by the results. Over one hundred spaces have been created in the past twelve years. While TKF was a funding partner in all these spaces, our contribution nearly always included a challenge grant. It is important to note that the dollars invested by others often exceeded our own, proof that the energy of the creating partnerships was contagious. In addition, an even greater contribution was the acquisition of the land itself. In most cases, it took the concerted effort of the creating partners and their kindred spirits to secure the land's ownership or use. The sweat and energy involved in planning the space, clearing the land, enriching the soil, and tangibly planting nature's elements created diverse and sustainable communities. The projects often blossomed into permanent public/private partnerships, ensuring commitment both to ongoing maintenance and to expanded programming.

Many of these projects have been carved out of the most unlikely of settings—from the violent, drug-addled city neighborhood to the high-security prison. This book is about a few of the many open spaces and sacred places that became a reality because of these leaders' vision and determination. We call these leaders, these creating partners, *Firesouls™,* because they are individuals who have the spark of hope and energy to find a way, often in the most challenging of circumstances, to foster the creation of places that can become sacred and embedded in nature. The Firesouls have been equally determined to make these sites open and welcoming to all.

As part of that outreach, there is a TKF-designed bench and a waterproof journal at every location, for visitors to stop and relax and share their experiences in writing. Over time, we have collected thousands of entries. People of all ages, races, religions, and nationalities have contributed. We know we are doing something right. We can see it affirmed in the sentiments expressed through the various journal entries. The visitors are experiencing the same fundamental transformation that Kitty and I felt in that park in London. They are bearing witness to the power of nature to heal and to unify. The experience of the creation and increasing use of these places has brought to TKF a body of experience and knowledge that can be utilized in the enhancement of those spaces that are to come.

It often strikes me that in a time of such unprecedented freedom in America, many of us feel trapped in lives of isolation and despair. This book is an antidote to that isolation. We hope to inform and inspire—and to remind each of you that in a time of increasing separation, even the smallest steps toward fostering community and introspection can yield incredible rewards. In the subsequent chapters, I will lead you on a tour of several places and show you the physical elements that go into shaping a sacred space. You will see excerpts from journal entries, which are personal revelations that speak to the power of these sites. *These journal entries appear in green in the margins throughout the book.* And you will hear, firsthand, from the people who were the driving force behind these projects. Co-author Carolyn Rapp interviewed the Firesouls and created a story for each that allows readers to glimpse the passion and determination of these individuals intent on helping us to discover our best possible selves.

—*Tom Stoner*

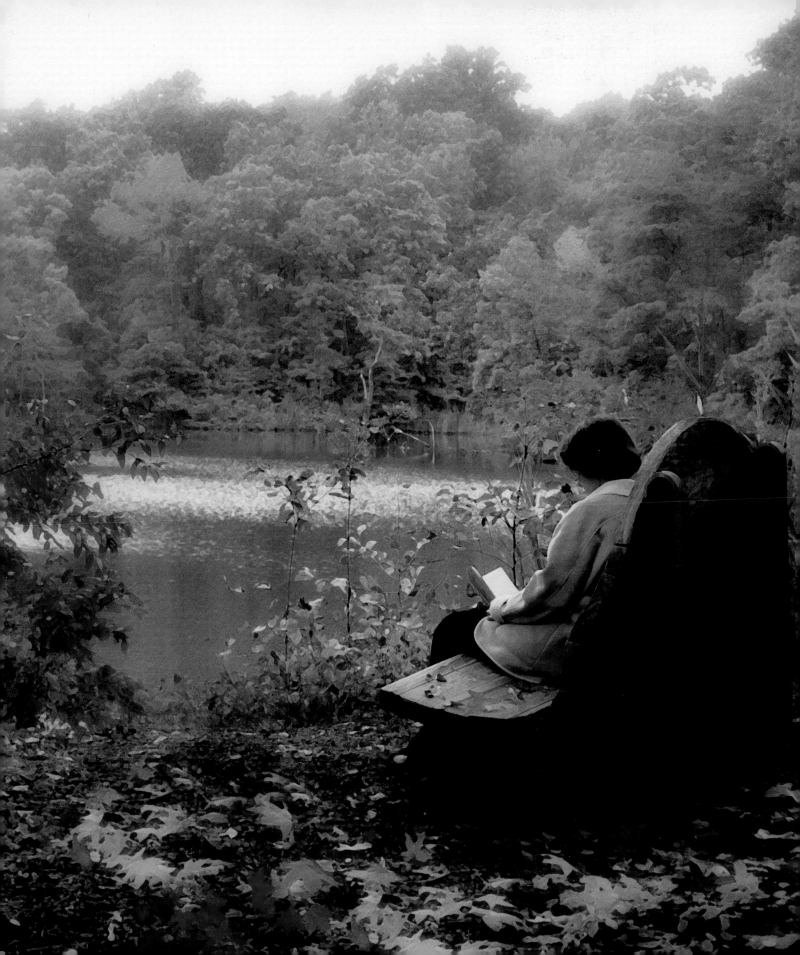

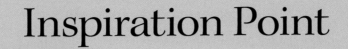

1 Inspiration Point

I believe that one Wow! experience can have the power to change the course of a person's life, because that's what happened to me.

—Don Baugh, Firesoul

Kitty and I arrived at the Chesapeake Bay the same way John Smith did back in 1607—we sailed in. The further we ventured up the Bay, the more it resonated with our natures. It has the vast expanse of the Boundary Waters that meant so much to me as a young man. And the life of the rivers and creeks that make up so much of the Bay area reminded Kitty of the movement of the waters of the Mississippi. We made it our home. And we made it the location of our very first TKF project ten years ago.

At the time, Will Baker, president of the Chesapeake Bay Foundation, a nonprofit organization founded in 1967 to help protect and restore this vast watershed, was leading the way in planning a new headquarters. The sustainable building would sit on thirty-three acres along the Bay, just outside Annapolis, Maryland. It would be the locus for environmental policy and change, but creating that change promised to be a conflict-ridden process. There are many different points of view about how to clean the Bay. It seemed important to create a refuge near the headquarters where people could retreat from heated discussions. By being in a place that centered them in nature,

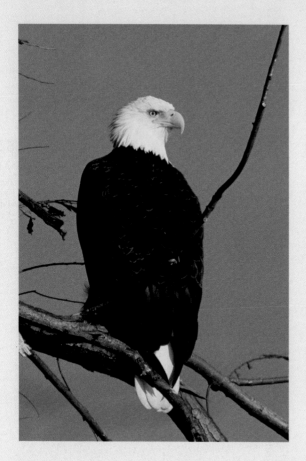

they would be more likely to mull over the opportunities and the difficulties of what they were doing and make sound decisions.

Picking this first location proved to be an amazing progression, antithetical to what I knew as the head of a media business. The planning process I had always followed was very traditional: set goals, construct structures that would support those goals, create incentives. But that's not the way the Chesapeake team operated. Its process was much more organic. Rather than choose a site along the considerable expanse of shoreline fronting the open waters of the Bay, the team chose a more remote spot overlooking a creek. They chose it because it was intimate, and because it was once the site of a Native American settlement. They chose it because, to this day, it is where the eagles nest.

Basing a site plan on the flying patterns of birds is definitely not something that would exist in a traditional business plan. But what emerged from this process was a new understanding about what *sacred* and *open* really mean. We didn't have a strict definition of these words going into this first project, and if we had, we would have been in trouble. We learned that a project like this has to emerge. The power has to come from the community; it has to be a collective, intuitive decision. You need open souls, and you need people who have no agenda. An architect once told me that an idea such as this is like a little flower. It's very delicate. You don't want to stamp on it.

The true wonder of the decision to place Inspiration Point along this secluded stretch of creek was that the team unanimously came to that decision. By kayaking and hiking through these many acres, by taking their own individual paths, they arrived at the same point. And we at TKF learned a valuable lesson: we learned to have faith that our grantees have the wisdom to know what's best. Inspiration Point didn't start in the design lab or in the boardroom; it started in the human heart. It started with a group of dedicated people following the flight path of an eagle. And with each subsequent TKF project, these open spaces sacred places emerge anew.

—*T.S.*

Don Baugh

Vice President of Education, Chesapeake Bay Foundation

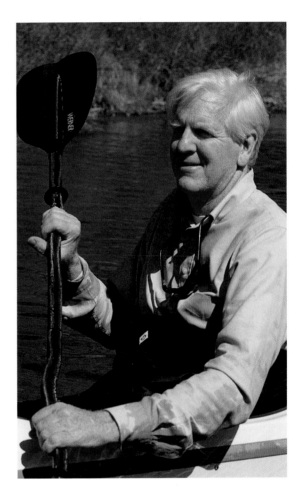

Liquid stillness—time floats by
Dusk descends with a hush.

I believe to my core that a single Wow! experience can have the power to change the course of a person's life, because that's what happened to me. Behind my dorm at college, there was a little stream. Nobody paid much attention to it, and people threw litter into it; but nature often manages to defend itself, and that stream became my place of reflection. Sitting on the bank, surrounded by trees and listening to the water, helped me figure out what I really wanted to do with my life. I changed my major from physics, which I was good at, to conservation, which I knew in my gut was what I really wanted to do. For the last thirty years, I've been helping people discover the world of the Chesapeake Bay and to see it as sacred.

I should define what *sacred* means to me. Everyone agrees that beauty is in the eye of the beholder, and I think that the definition of *sacred* also depends on the individual's view. For me, it has nothing to do with religion or belief or creed. It has to do with a connection, a feeling that makes me sure that there is something more powerful going on than what I can see. I feel that connection at many places in the Bay. With its hundreds of miles of shoreline and its countless creeks, rivers, coves, and ponds, there are hundreds of little intimate places where one can sit and feel connections that are stronger than the five senses. I'm sure others would agree with me. The Chesapeake Bay is not designated a national shrine, but many people who spend time on the Bay develop a deep, strong connection with this landscape. For me, *sacred* is the word that describes that connection.

When the TKF Foundation decided that it wanted to create its first sacred spaces around the Chesapeake Bay, I was given the task of putting together a committee to choose the sites. That was easy. So many people's lives have been touched and changed by their experiences on the Bay that I quickly assembled an enthusiastic group that included board members, naturalists, a photographer, a writer, and others.

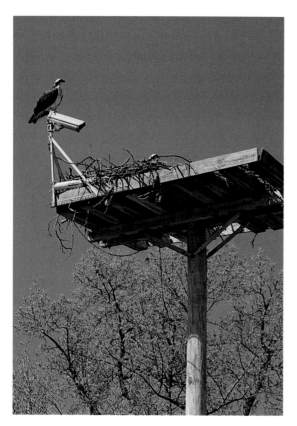

But the Bay is enormous, so before the whole committee went searching, I made a list of places for them to visit. To help me figure out which of the many inspirational, spiritual places I would take the committee to visit, I chose a couple of filters. The first was the sites of Native American villages. For more than ten thousand years before the European settlers arrived, Native Americans lived in the Chesapeake Bay area. They had their choice of where to establish their villages, and it seemed to me they always chose special places—often near rivers, streams, or freshwater springs, commonly on the rise of a hill that afforded a view, generally near forests that provided shelter and hunting, and near the Bay for food—fish, oysters, crabs, and clams.

My second lens was the locations of bald eagles' nests, because eagles have their choice of sites as well. Bald eagles were near extinction in the late 1970s, but thanks to protective laws, improved water quality, and good wildlife management policies, the bald eagle has made a comeback to more than nine hundred nesting pairs in the Chesapeake Bay region. Eagles choose the tallest trees in quiet, natural places that are surrounded by a certain amount of open space—just the qualities we were looking for in our sacred places.

I came up with the list, and the committee went looking—by boat, by canoe, by foot. When they saw the site here at the headquarters building—which wasn't yet built at the time—there was unanimous agreement. Actually,

The ospreys are very active today. What a delicate chirp from such a big bird. One splashed down directly in front of me and caught a nice white perch. Thoughts of the office grind and the headlines on Iraq sort of drift away on this sacred bench.
Thank you.

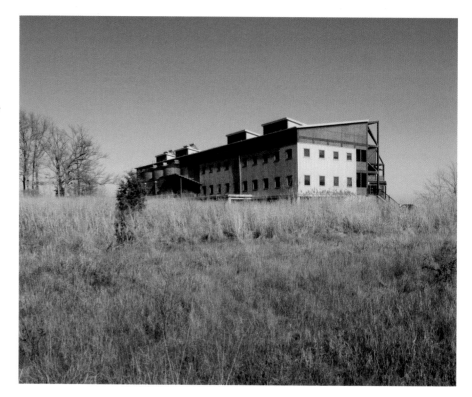

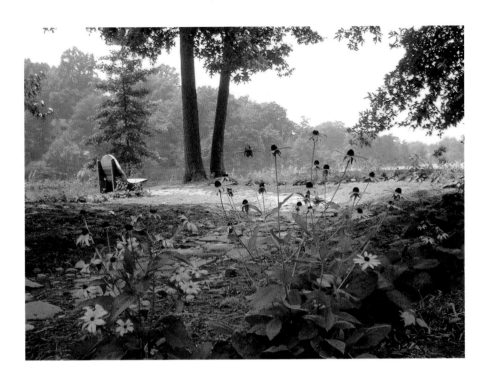

it was not an easy call because there are a number of lovely places on this property. But when people got to this particular site, we all realized that we had reached the end of our search. It just felt right, and that was it. It was Inspiration Point. We later designated three more sacred sites around the Bay, all at places where we have educational centers—Fox Island, Smith Island, and Bishop's Head. We made a conscious decision to do this because it ensured that many people would discover the sites through our educational programs.

The Chesapeake Bay Foundation is in the business of connecting people to nature. While we do this through teaching them about the Bay and taking them out to do field investigation, we also foster the connection in another way. We try to expose our participants, many of whom are children, to places that are so beautiful and so unforgettable that their jaws just drop open and they say, "Wow! Is this amazing or what!" I call that the Wow! factor.

Each of our educational centers was built on a Wow! factor site. It made perfect sense to look there for our sacred sites and to put benches and journals there, because our programs always include time for reflection and expression. We now use all of the sacred sites as focal points for our programs, for both children and adults. I've watched their faces as they see a heron spread its enormous wings and take flight or an osprey dive for its prey or a fiery sun set over the water. I've read what they write in the bench journals that tell me they truly "get" the sacred connection between us and the environment we live in. And I feel hopeful about the future of the Bay.

This is the most healing place I know. When I gaze at the water, the steady wave of currents reminds me that the peace I feel is eternal. I listen to the trees say "shhhhhhh" and I trust the quietness. I feel my hair brush my face, and I realize how affected I am by things I can't even see, things greater than me.

I hope someday to be married on this beautiful point of land.

If this bench could talk

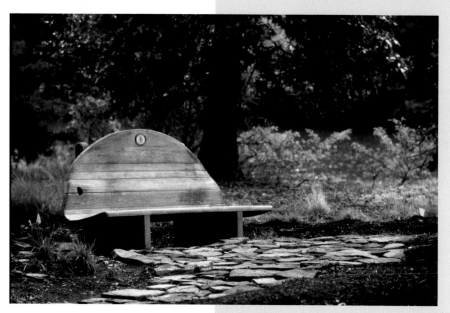

I come from the long ago. I'm not really sure how old I am. I remember Indian camps, dusty roads, ox carts, horses, wagons, stagecoaches, and travelers on foot. About 1890 or so it was, so I am told, when I was cut down at last—"virgin timber," they called me. Seemed to prize me greatly, declaring me "just right." Not until later did I learn that only certain extremely tight-grain trees—such as fir, cypress, redwood, and pine—were considered good enough for pickle barrels.

They put me to work in a pickle factory, filled with pickles and pickle brine. You'd be amazed how popular I was! Time passed and I was emptied, dried out, and rudely left to rot. But I didn't. Horseless carriages chugged by, cars whizzed by, and much later, jet planes screamed far overhead, leaving cloudy trails behind.

I truly thought my life was done, but not so. About a hundred years after I was first filled with pickles, I was picked up and hauled in a truck to a small carpenter shop on Maryland's Eastern Shore. This time my destiny was to become a bench. But not just any bench—no indeed! Rather, one lovingly created by my craftsmen and an architect, of all things! I was intended to retain the natural roundness of the barrel I had been for so long. Even the staves came along: they were fashioned into legs.

Some day I hope to have the strength and serenity of a pickle barrel. May this place and this bench grant me that strength. May God grant me the serenity.

So here I am, in this beautiful place. Serene, isn't it? A place in which to dream, to meditate, to recover from stress and trauma, a place in which to reconnect. Lean back, stranger, and rest. In me is the strength of half a millennium; permit me to share it with you. But in me too is peace and tranquility.

Do not leave me until that strength and peace come to you. And when you do leave me, don't stay away long.

I'll be here, waiting for you—in this sacred place.

Chuck Foster

Chief of Staff, Chesapeake Bay Foundation

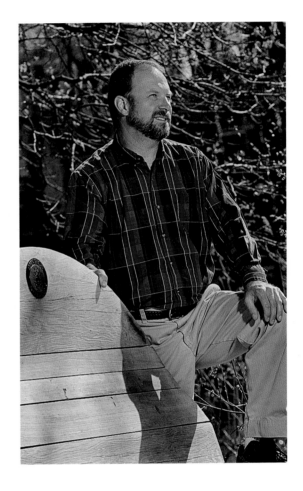

My role in this project was very straightforward: I was the bench builder. Once Don Baugh and the committee members had chosen the site for Inspiration Point, TKF decided that they would like to place a bench that would invite people to sit and reflect and be restored by the beauty of the Bay. Don came to me and said, "We're considering commercial benches, but I know you can do better. Can you come up with a design?" So Don, his wife, Janet Harrison, who is an architect, my co-worker Paul Willey, and I sat down and talked about what a bench in a sacred place should look like.

At that time, we had access to some pickle vats from an old plant in Marydale, Maryland—and I have to make it clear that I'm talking about pickle vats, not pickle barrels. These old pickling vats were swimming pool size—more than eight feet high and fourteen to sixteen feet in diameter. They were built specifically for pickle factories, and the wood was just beautiful. All of it was old growth, some of it redwood, and all of it was pickled so that the pores were very tight. The four of us agreed that giving this old wood a new life would be a wonderful thing, as well as a metaphor for the kind of revitalization that TKF was hoping to engender in people who visited these sacred sites. We wanted to keep as much of the original quality of the vats as possible, which is why the design included rounded edges and curves, echoing the curves of the vats. We also wanted a bench that invited community, so we made it big enough for five or six people.

When I built the first bench, TKF liked it so much that it became their signature bench. They wanted one at each of their gardens. But that presented us with the huge challenge of locating enough wood to make dozens of benches. When we ran out of the wood from the Maryland plant, we started research-ing. We found a plant in North Carolina that was going out of business. Paul and I flew down there to check out the vats and arranged to have them

I will tell you why I love this place. I love this place because no matter where I go I can take it with me. No matter what.

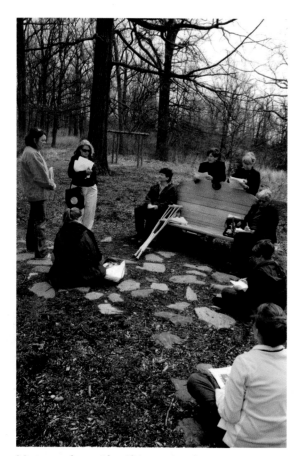

Master gardeners identifying native plants

shipped back. That kept us in wood for a while, but we knew we couldn't keep flying around the country looking for pickle vats. Fortunately, we found a man in Chicago who did the traveling himself and salvaged the old wood. I went out and trained him to build the benches, and he supplied us with the next round of benches. Then we discovered that we could have them built through the Maryland prison system, and that took the metaphor one step further—prisoners, who were hopefully in a redemption mode, redeeming this old wood and rebirthing it into new benches.

To get to that first bench we built for Inspiration Point, visitors encounter three of the basic elements of a sacred space—a path that leads to the space, a portal to pass through, and an altar. Our path is made of fine gravel that is earth-friendly in that it allows water to seep into the ground. It also meets the American Disability Act requirements so that the space is accessible to all. The path leads to a portal that takes visitors out to a lovely wooded site overlooking the Bay.

Ironically, the portal was installed on September 11, 2001. It had arrived at headquarters, but we hadn't set an installation date. Of course, on September 11, everyone here at work was glued to the television all morning, watching those awful images along with the rest of the world. At about noon, we decided to go out to Inspiration Point and install the portal. It gave us a way to turn away from the terrible destruction of that day and focus on all that is possible if we can find peace in our hearts and work out of that. The portal will always have a special meaning for me because of that day.

I used to hate life—so much as to end it.
I thank the Lord I am still here. Look up!
How can you not love this place?

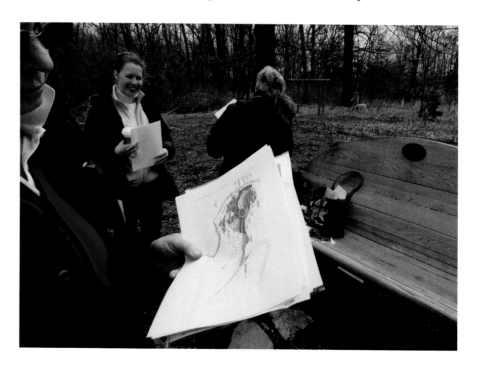

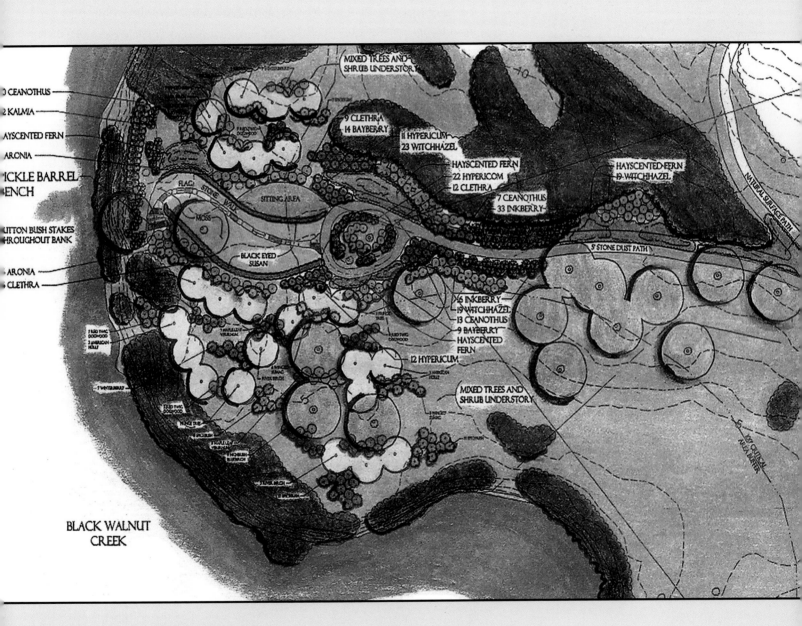

MIXED TREES AND
SHRUB UNDERSTORY

9 CLETHRA
14 BAYBERRY

11 HYPERICUM
23 WITCHHAZEL

HAYSCENTED FERN
22 HYPERICUM
12 CLETHRA

HAYSCENTED FERN
19 WITCHHAZEL

7 CEANOTHUS
33 INKBERRY

3 CEANOTHUS

2 KALMIA

HAYSCENTED FERN

ARONIA

ICKLE BARREL
ENCH

UTTON BUSH STAKES
HROUGHOUT BANK

ARONIA

CLETHRA

FLAG STONE WALL

SITTING AREA

MOSS

BLACK EYED
SUSAN

5 STONE DUST PATH

NATURAL SURFACE PATH

16 INKBERRY
19 WITCHHAZEL
13 CEANOTHUS
9 BAYBERRY
HAYSCENTED
FERN

12 HYPERICUM

MIXED TREES AND
SHRUB UNDERSTORY

BLACK WALNUT
CREEK

We know that many people use the benches for meditation—people who live nearby, visitors to the islands, and both adults and children in our education programs. We know because of what they write in the journals. But when we came up with the first design for the bench, it didn't include the concept of a journal. Early on in this project, I mentioned to my mother what I was involved in. Shortly after that, she sent me a magazine article about a bench in a mountain setting, which had a journal attached to it. It was an immediate "Aha!" experience for all of us. We modified the design to include a slot beneath the bench where a waterproof journal could be kept. I think the journals elevate this whole project because they provide a way to gain insight into the people who visit the spaces. Without that feedback, the people at TKF could put in a space and eventually forget about it, as they move on to other projects. But the journals provide daily feedback from the people who use the spaces, and that feedback keeps each space alive. It gives us the feeling that we are having an impact on both individual lives and society.

So, yes, I built the benches for the sacred space here at the Chesapeake Bay Foundation and for a number of other sites. But the story goes beyond the benches. The story is really about sacred spaces that have the power to restore our souls and transform our lives, and about the people who use those spaces and go back into the world more peaceful, more inspired, more whole.

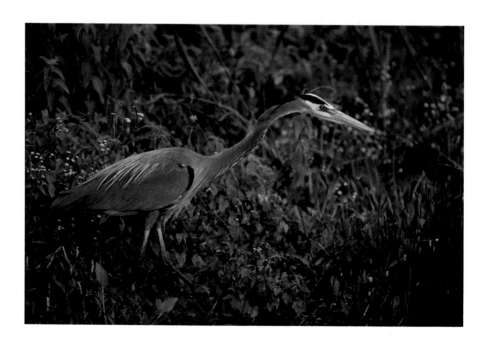

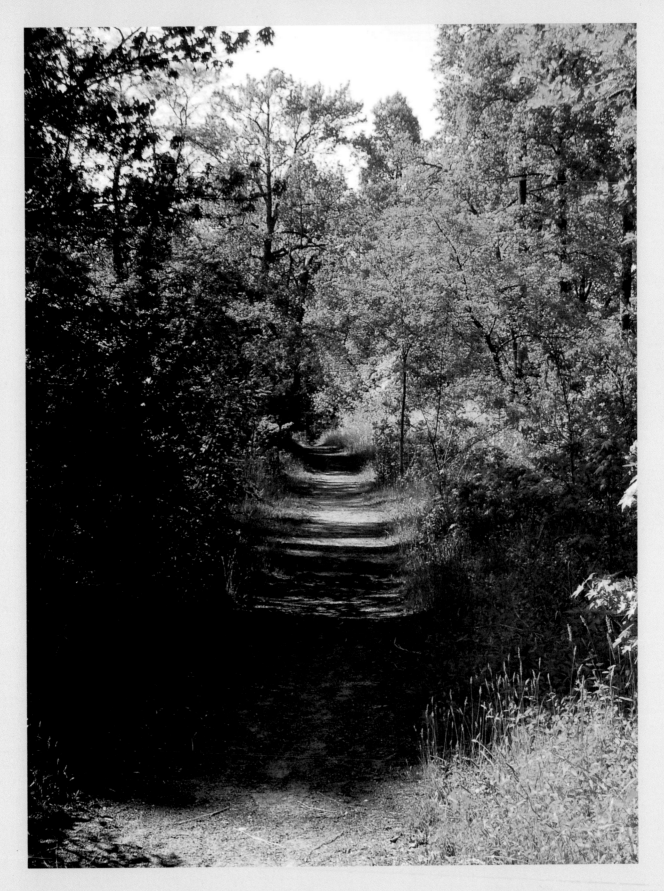

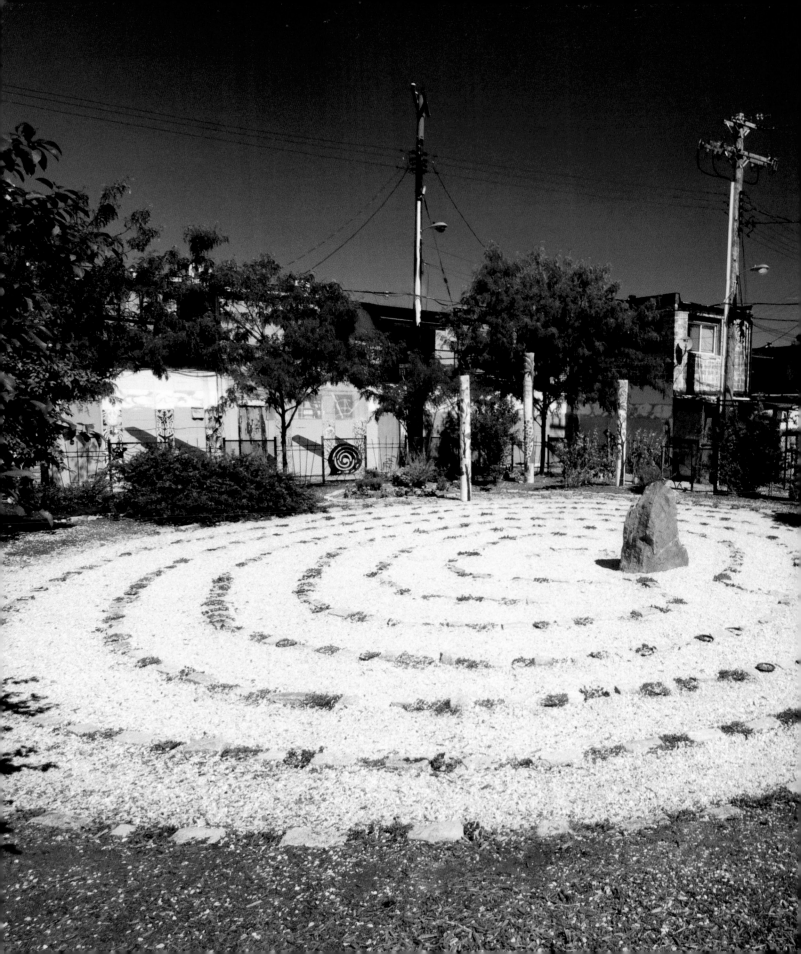

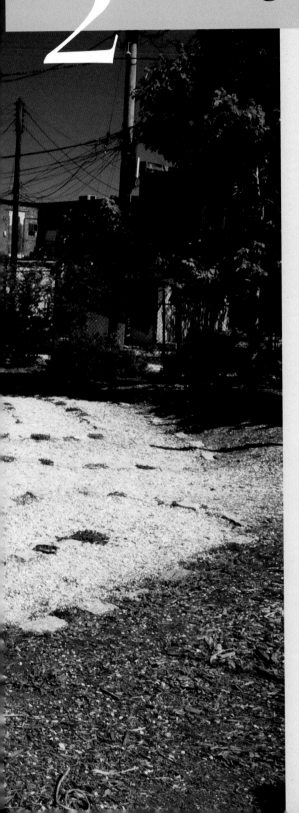

2 Amazing Port Street Sacred Commons

*On one side of the fence, a guy was
selling crack; on the other, people just
kept building the labyrinth.*

—Jerry Waters, Firesoul

For an accessible sacred place to exist, it must be protected by a sense
of surround, or a zone of safety, that can be felt by all. This is especially
important in an urban setting like the McElderry Park neighborhood.
Situated in a city with nearly three hundred murders each year, McElderry
Park in East Baltimore tops the list of violent places. Once a thriving family
community, it devolved over the decades; today, the corners belong to the
drug dealers. Empty lots and abandoned homes are rat-infested dumping
grounds, and too many of the young men who roam the streets wind up
statistics in the police blotter.

In 1999, Karen Brau, the pastor of Amazing Grace Evangelical Lutheran
Church on McElderry Street, had the vision to create a haven in the midst
of this blight. Karen's early training in economics gave her the organiza-
tional skills she needed to nurture an enduring partnership between the
church and the neighborhood community association. Karen and one of the
community association's leaders, Jerry Waters, worked together to galvanize
the community to turn a number of abandoned lots behind the church into
a small garden. They later added a labyrinth, and Karen took to its path
every day to walk among the gangs and the dealers. She aimed to take back

her neighborhood one step at a time. Inspired by her courage, Jerry asked dangerous intruders to leave. Over time, they created a distinct zone of safety, an understood division between the violence of the neighborhood and the peace within the labyrinth. They slowly pushed back the forces of decay, poverty, crime, and fear.

Today, the ripple effect of what they helped build is being felt throughout the neighborhood, as more and more residents join to repair the community from within. This place once known for chaos and crime is now where the community can gather among flowers and shrubs to celebrate, to mourn, and to believe in their own ability to be transformed through peace and hope. Through their force of character, constancy, and quest to build community, Karen and Jerry inspired the neighborhood to create this green refuge called Amazing Port Street Sacred Commons. It is truly as amazing as its name.

—T.S.

No matter where we go in the world, no matter how much "progress" our society achieves, we will always need open places filled with nature that let us recharge our soul and see the world in a fresh light.

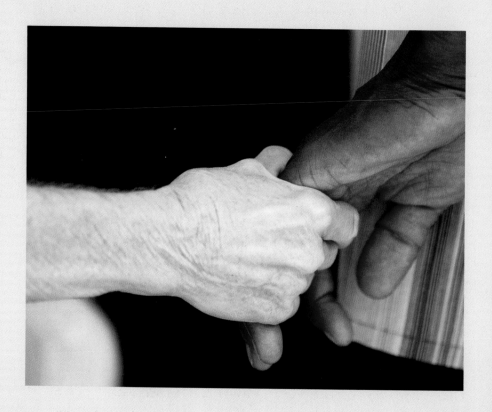

Karen Brau

Pastor, Amazing Grace Evangelical Lutheran Church

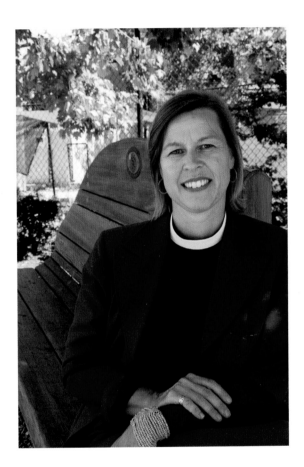

My father is a Lutheran pastor, my grandfather was a Lutheran pastor, and I was determined to be anything but a Lutheran pastor. So I went to college, where I majored in economics, and then I worked in New York City at a large commercial bank. The training program was excellent, and I did so well that the senior management wanted to send me to Columbia University for a master of business administration degree. With my foot practically on the threshold to begin the MBA, something started working inside of me, and I just couldn't do it. It didn't feel right. I made a 180-degree turn and started exploring possibilities for working within a church structure. I ended up going to seminary in Louisville, Kentucky, where I developed a passion for urban ministry. The scriptures are filled with references to justice, and the prophets speak a lot about living out justice in the world. I was drawn to that and was fortunate to work with some African American women who taught me what that could mean. That's how I found my way to the McElderry Park community of East Baltimore. I've been serving this neighborhood since 1990.

Drug addiction is a huge problem in this community. Almost every household has some member of the family actively addicted, and it affects everything—the economy, the level of anxiety in the community, people's ability to leave their houses, and, of course, the children. Along with the drugs come drug dealers and gangs—and gang violence. When someone gets shot, it has a ripple effect of negative energy on the family and friends, and then on the whole community. That's our reality, and yet in the midst of all this, I think we've done some very encouraging things.

For example, we have heard from several sources that one day this summer, about fifteen members of a local gang came to the labyrinth we built on

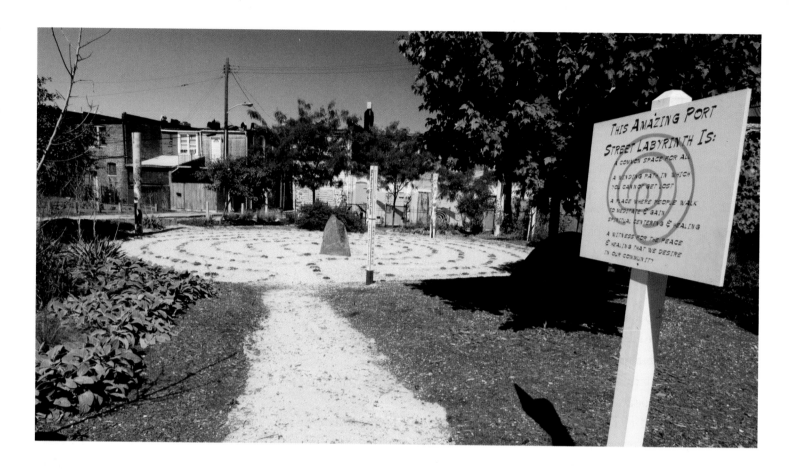

I experience the labyrinth as simply a map, a circuitous slow walk from the first step on the perimeter into the very center... It honors a need for introspection and stillness. It is a place to acknowledge illness and healing, death and birth and pain, a place to face fear, listen for an inner voice, seek hope or faith or perhaps take a breath.

Amazing Port Street, behind the church. A neighbor was concerned, so she watched. The young men just sat in the labyrinth. After a while, they left. We later learned that one of the members of their gang had been shot—and their response was to come to the labyrinth. Now, there probably isn't one among them who would set foot in a church. It's not that they are not welcomed by me; it's that their whole perception is that the Church would not welcome them. I've been here long enough to know that no matter how much outreach you do, some people are just not going to come inside. Yet these kids knew—they felt on some level—that the labyrinth was sacred space, and in their suffering, they came to it. To me, that's the whole vision of the Church. I believe that everyone has a longing for the holy, and whether they have access to it or not could be one of those turning points in life—a moment when they can be touched by something that is outside of their immediate suffering and change becomes possible. That's what our labyrinth is: accessible sacred space.

The greening and beautification of the area behind our church that eventually led to the creation of the labyrinth began with a garden. I love gardening and learned how to take care of a garden when I was growing up. When I decided that I was going to stay here for a while, I needed something that linked my passion to a concrete activity that would engage others as well. Our first garden was created by the children of the church, and it was wonderful. It also gave me the opportunity to teach them what a garden means, and for me, it means preparation and nurturing and ongoing attending. Then finally, it's about results. Our results have been flowers and varying levels of produce.

In 1999, we learned that the City was going to tear down the houses on both sides of the narrow street that runs alongside of and behind the church. Our block was in a designated empowerment zone, and there was government money to demolish the houses and rework the space. The houses did come down, but there was no plan for redoing the space. Then—who knows how—the money for the project was gone, and there was nothing there but an empty, ugly, rubble-strewn space, which became a magnet for drug dealers and users. There was some talk of a private development plan for creating some greenspace, and we looked at some possibilities. I have a friend who is involved in labyrinths, and she suggested putting one in the Port Street space. We even worked with some architecture students from a nearby university on a plan that included a labyrinth, but in the end, that design was not feasible. In the meantime, for the two summers while we were in limbo, the kids in the church summer camp created small labyrinths out of rubble and found objects.

Finally, it became apparent that if anything was going to get done, it was going to get done through this church in partnership with the community, which is represented by the McElderry Park Community Association. I've done a lot of community organizing, and for the outcome to be authentic, you have to pay attention to the place and to the people in it, even if they're not part of the church. Besides being the right thing to do, I knew that by partnering with the community association, we could leverage resources in a way that would benefit the overall project. A faith-based institution has one set of resources, and a community association has another set. I took one of the women in my congregation aside and said, "There's something we want to do. Who do I have to know in the community association?" She said, "Jerry Waters," and she invited the two of us over to her house to talk. After I did a little explaining about this "weird" idea of a labyrinth, Jerry jumped wholeheartedly on board and did a huge amount of the work that made it a reality.

To me, faith has to do with healing. The practice of walking a labyrinth combines the two, faith and healing. Faith-healing doesn't mean that things are perfect, but rather that wounds can be healed in the context of faith, and sometimes those wounds become gifts. For example, there is a woman in the neighborhood who was an addict for a long time, and her heart had grown hard. But I kept pushing her to become involved and engaged. By being part

Just for today I am grateful for being alive. I am blessed to be able to think clearly without the use of a drug regulating my mind. Thank you, God, for your many blessings and for your strength to make it through this day.

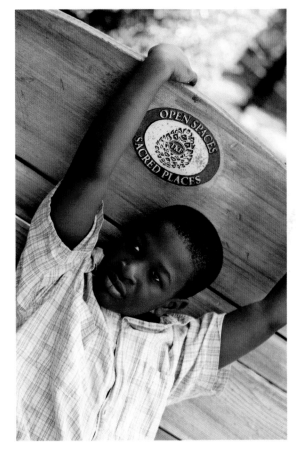

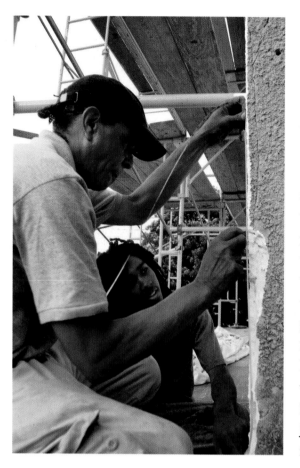

I try to remember to breathe, to stay focused, to not run from my fears, to stay connected. It is new, it is interesting, it is scary, and ultimately it is all right. I am still me, trying my best, looking for goodness in the world.

of a group that talked about faith, she has moved into recovery and become alive in ways that surprise even her. She is beginning to see fruit in her life that she never imagined possible, and she is becoming an authentic voice that faith is alive. There are other stories and things happening in our neighborhood that point to the healing that is beginning to take place, and I thought that the labyrinth could be a part of that. I hoped it would serve as a reminder that there is something greater than ourselves; that no matter what, love can't be obliterated. I hoped that the labyrinth would be a powerful witness of hope and healing for this neighborhood. And, in fact, it has.

When we started, dealers were selling drugs, and junkies were shooting up there every night. Each day, before we could allow volunteers to start their work building the labyrinth, Jerry and a couple of others had to walk the property to pick up used syringes, so that no one would inadvertently stick themselves with a needle. We finished the labyrinth in 2001, and in 2002, I took a sabbatical leave. When I returned, the drug dealers were still all over the place. I decided that I was going to bear witness. Part of dealing with the problem was calling the police, but another part was what my faith required of me: stepping out there and putting myself on the line for the vision I had. So I walked the labyrinth for a year—not every single day, but at least four days a week. I would walk, and the dealers would be just outside the labyrinth, selling their drugs. But today, they aren't there. The walking, the being there, and Jerry talking to them, telling them they needed to move on—it has made a difference. The word is out to leave that space alone.

I also think that just seeing the Amazing Port Street project come to completion has been very healing for the neighborhood, because it proves that things can get done. Cities make lots of promises about what they're going to do for urban neighborhoods, and very often nothing happens. That experience has led to a high level of disgust and distrust and disconnection among the people who live in those neighborhoods. This project was developed and completed as a result of the community and church working together, and that is a powerful demonstration of this neighborhood's possibilities.

This whole space has been conducive to an unfolding of beauty, which I think is such an important piece in touching the deepest place in a person. First, the garden. Then, the labyrinths the children made. Then, the permanent labyrinth. While all this was going on, the McElderry Park Community Association received, as a gift, a house and a piece of land that is across the street from the labyrinth. We've turned that land into greenspace for the community—a lawn and a flower garden with marigolds planted in the shape of the word *love*. The City brought pieces of telephone poles and planted them

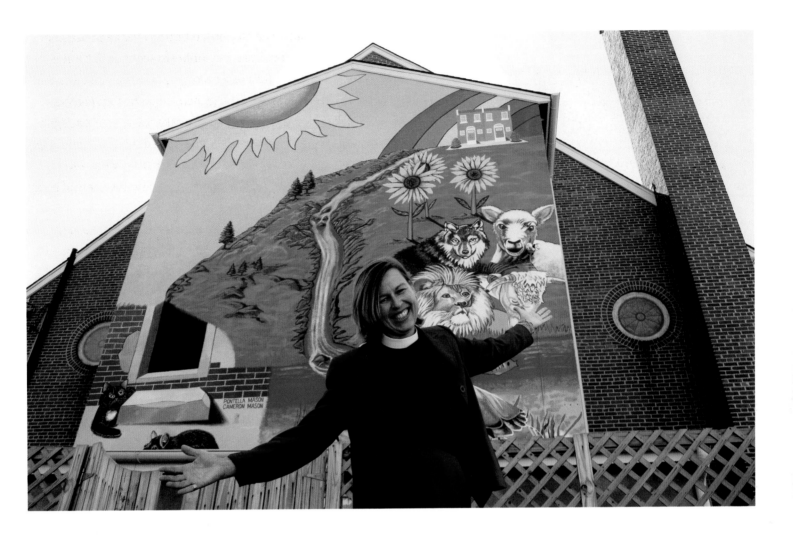

around the labyrinth, and the children made them into painted totem poles. The TKF Foundation, which funded the labyrinth, also funded the fence, which is not closed fencing, but simply defines the space and sets it off as different and sacred. We received money from another foundation to paint murals on the backs of the stores next to the labyrinth. They also funded a wonderful colorful sign that says "Amazing Port Street."

Most recently, an artist completed the mural that covers the back wall of the church. In conceiving the design, we used a text from Isaiah. To describe what peace looks like, Isaiah uses images of animals together that are not supposed to get along—the lion and the lamb, the cattle and the wolf. We had an artist work with us to interpret this passage from an urban vantage point. At the bottom of the mural are the predominant urban animals—the rat, roach, and cat—and a house in disrepair. Then the text talks about God's holy mountain, where the living water will flow, everyone will know God, and all creatures will get along. We took those elements of transformation and tried

It is NEVER too late to try your best!
NEVER too late to smile.
NEVER too late to forgive.
NEVER too late to try again, and when you do,
It just might be AMAZING.

I see you across the way, walking your own path, the same path, my path.

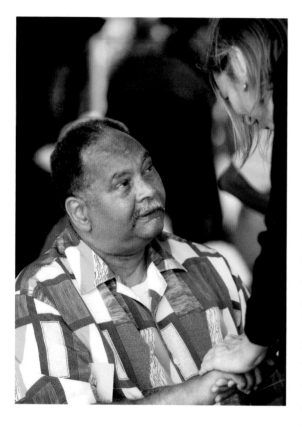

It is only in taking the first step that the path begins to unfold.

to bring them to life. The mural is so vibrant that it calms the area around the labyrinth and helps to form the sense of surround that is so important to a sacred space. There is no mistaking that behind the church is a very different space than the street in front of the church. Now we have more community events outside, and more people are participating. We've expanded from Sunday worship and a celebration of the space with refreshments to some evening events, and we've partnered with an operation named Safe Streets, an initiative supported by the health department, which reaches out to young people, teaching nonviolence.

As a person of faith, I believe it is the Holy Spirit that enables us to experience what peace is—and peace is not necessarily quiet. It's not necessarily that image of sheep lying placidly in a field. Peace can have a lot of moving parts, where all are engaging in what they do really well. For example, at an evening event in the Sacred Commons, young men were performing hip-hop and rap, and there was a strong connection between them and the audience. I believe that if we can offer this physical space and space enough within ourselves, as church and community, to create these possibilities that may seem impossible in an inner city neighborhood, then we smash the stereotypes that keep people stuck. When we turn things over, I think we're doing exactly what Jesus would do. The expectation is that there are certain limits to what we can do. But I think Jesus would say, "No, there's more, because the Kingdom of God turns things over."

I think that's what we are beginning to see, and while it's very exciting, there are still days when I feel overwhelmed by the enormity of the task and the relatively small steps we've taken. I've done funerals for young black men, and each one is a test for me. I did a funeral for the grandson of a member of this congregation, a very affable young man who was the wrong target of someone's bullet. I will never forget that funeral. As pastor, I escort the coffin to where it is going to be placed into the ground. That day, I turned and looked back, and there was a river of young black men and women following me to the grave. It was just so wrenching, because this young man didn't have to die. The heavy, toxic notion of a senseless death and the feeling of helplessness tested my faith. But often, at moments like these when I feel the absence of God and I'm not getting answers, something unexpected happens to keep me going.

I remember vividly the day that the TKF Foundation took a busload of people to visit some of the labyrinths they had funded throughout this area, including ours. It was the year that I was walking the labyrinth, and I told the people about the drug dealing that was still going on at the time. They kept telling me how beautiful our labyrinth was, even though it wasn't as neat as

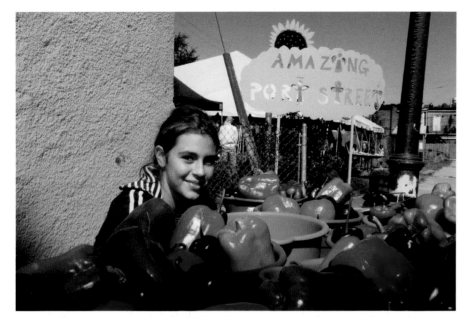

Spring has arrived to push back the veil of lingering frost. Let my heart awaken to new possibilities, let my soul shed its cocoon and struggle forth to unfold its magnificent wings and to fly, to soar, to flutter away.

others they had seen and its design not as perfect. In a neighborhood with a lot of vacant, boarded-up houses, in the midst of all this ruin and struggle, they had a visceral response: here is this Amazing Port Street Sacred Commons, and it's real. I think it was the depth of the space that embraced those people. It was pouring rain, but they walked the labyrinth anyway. Afterward, one of the women came up to me and said, "It rains on the just and the unjust." I loved that, because it was her way of expressing the conclusion I've come to, which is that good and evil coexist. You always trust that the love and the good are going to prevail, but evil keeps showing up too, and part of maturing on the journey of faith is to know that. Visitors often say, "It's awful that these drug dealers are here." And I would think to myself, "I don't know if it's awful, but it is real. And our labyrinth is real. And that's the world."

I love all things God has created, but that does not mean I have to like all of them.

The wonder of the labyrinth and the Amazing Port Street Sacred Commons project is that it has allowed something radical to come to life in our community. The labyrinth is also hugely important to me personally, offering a spiritual practice that not only keeps me grounded but also continually teaches me. As I walk the labyrinth, I am constantly reminded that everything goes to the center. Even the situations that cause me despair, cause me self-doubt, cause me to grieve and mourn and fight with God are parts of the journey, and the love of God is stronger than any of those feelings or realities. Love is the center and keeps pulling me toward it. It's vitally important to have a place where I feel that and know that, because what we are doing here is hard and profound work. We are transforming this neighborhood in the face of what seems impossible. And we're not giving up.

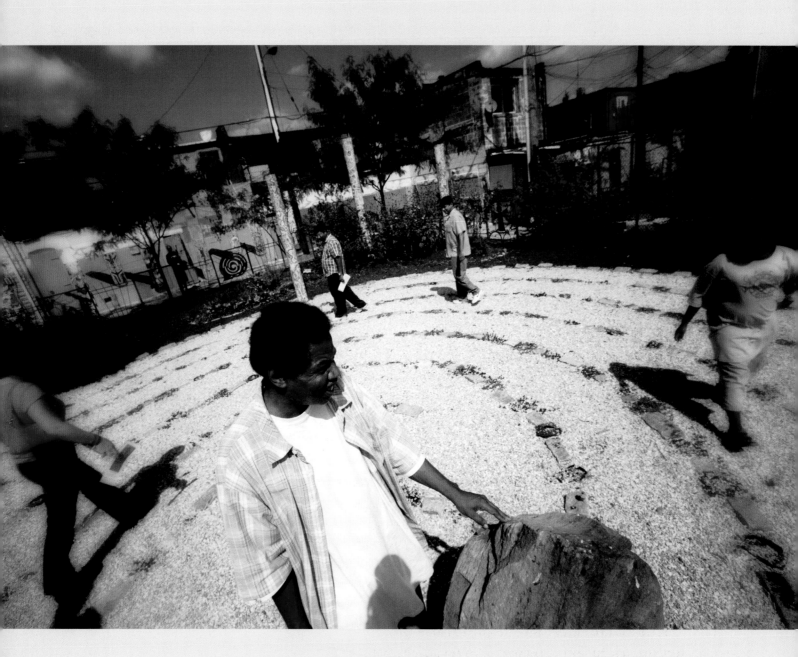

Jerry Waters

President, McElderry Park Community Association

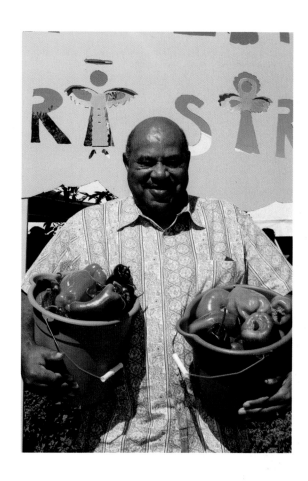

When I moved here twenty-five years ago, this was a different kind of neighborhood. For one thing, it was mixed, with black and white people living together. The streets didn't have trash on them, people could sit on their front steps and feel safe, and kids could play outside without parents worrying about shootings. But as people got older, they moved out and sold their houses. We started losing homeowners and gaining renters and transients. Then the businesses started leaving, and most of the landlords that bought the houses were interested only in collecting rent money. The neighborhood started to decline, with drugs and gangs affecting the safety and quality of life. My wife and I could have left, but I think that no matter where any of us go, we're going to find problems. And we can't keep running, or nothing will get solved. We have to make a stand somewhere, and I decided to make mine here.

And just look at Amazing Port Street now. Look at how far we've come. The crime rate is up in the rest of the city but down in McElderry Park. We used to have to pick up the syringes before we could work in the commons area; now the drug dealers stay away. And some of the same people who used to throw trash are now the people picking up the trash, sitting on the benches, walking the labyrinth, and using the space. It just goes to show that with the community and the church working together, good things can happen.

Part of our success has to do with Pastor Karen. We have a lot of churches that are *in* the community but not *part of* the community. But nobody can say that about Amazing Grace. It has a lot to do with the community. Pastor Karen is always visible: she doesn't just come to work and go home. I think because people knew that Pastor Karen was there and that the church was trying to do something good for the community, it made it easier to get them to work on the Amazing Port Street project and helped

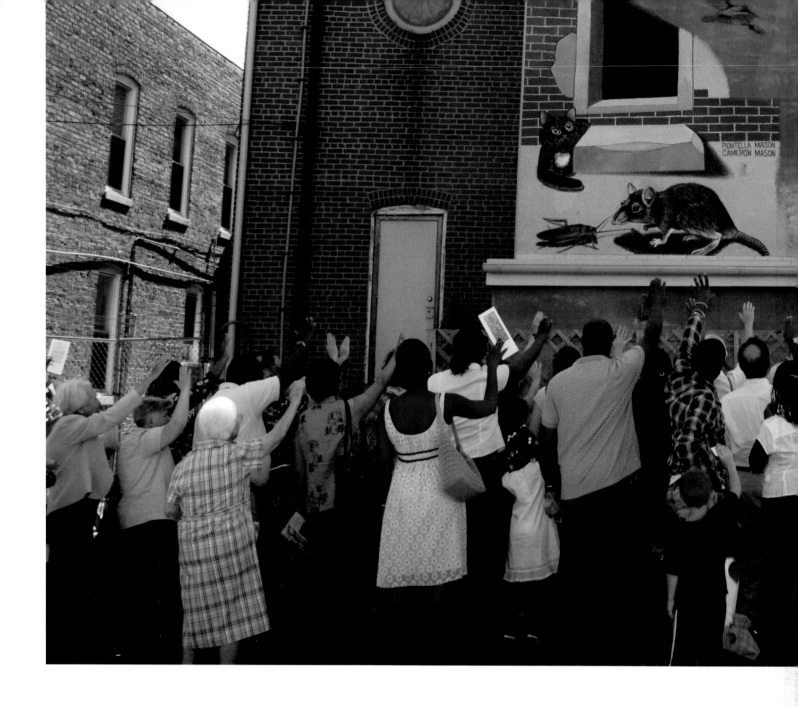

make it successful. The working relationship was never "yours" or "mine." It was always, "What can we do together?" And this wasn't one of those projects where one or the other of us said, "This is what we're going to do." We had meeting after meeting after meeting to decide what we were going to do with the land behind the church, until everybody was happy with the plan.

We built the labyrinth ourselves. We wanted to build it ourselves, because we wanted to get people involved. The main players were James Wooten and myself—we were there every day. My wife's the gardener of the family, and

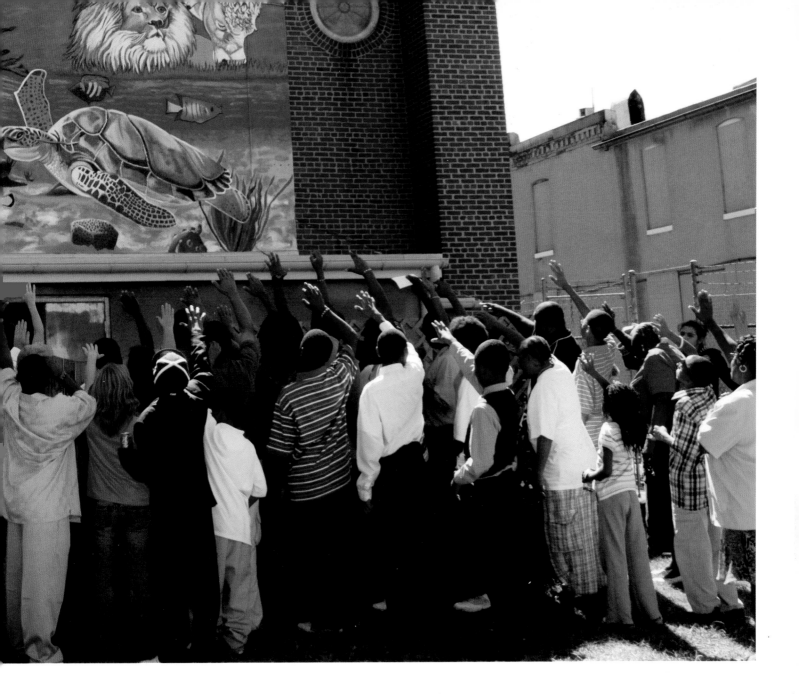

anyone who knows me will say I'm not much of a "dirt person." But Pastor Karen had me out there doing the dirty work on the labyrinth—from digging to laying stones in the hot sun. I believe that when people make a commitment to something, they should stick to it. And I have to say I got a lot of enjoyment out of this project.

One of the things that amazed me the most was how many people were willing to help. It was an intergenerational project for the community—men, women, teens, families, little children. It was so important to have the children

Now there is something to fear... our soul's desires not realized because we pandered to fear ... All we perhaps have to do is make the simple (and yes, perhaps brave) decision to serve beauty and to only wink at fear.

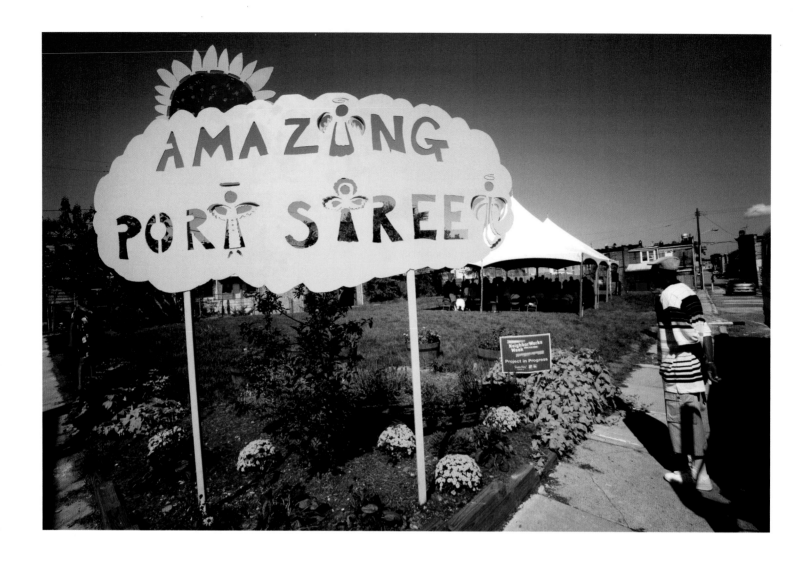

The way home to truth and peace is inward. Through the chaos. Beyond the stillness. In the innermost inner self. This is where God waits—inside of each one.

there that we found things for them to do. But the effort went far beyond the neighborhood. We asked for volunteers, and they appeared. People came from all over: we had volunteers from the United Way and a couple from Australia. One day, some sailors from a submarine that was docked in the harbor came over and worked all day. Another day, a whole busload of people pulled up and jumped out. "What do you want me to do? What do you want me to do?" they all were asking. That was just amazing to me. People hear about East Baltimore, and some panic just thinking about coming here, but volunteers came from all over the city. On one side of the fence, a guy was selling crack; on the other, people just kept on building the labyrinth. People took to the idea, and they came and helped.

While we were working on the labyrinth, a great thing happened for the neighborhood. There was a building that the McElderry Park Community

Association had wanted to buy for a long time, but its owner, Mr. Tudor, hadn't wanted to sell. The house had been in his family for a long time, and even though he didn't live in it, he used it for storage. Every so often, he and his wife would come down and go through their things. Then one day when they visited, he got robbed—and I just happened to walk up and stop the robbery. That's how we got connected. From then on, every time he and his wife came to the house, he would call me first and ask me to watch out for them. I'd sit in front of the house while he and his wife sorted through their things. He'd say, "Just fifteen minutes, Jerry." And it would turn out to be two or three hours, but I'd wait for him.

Then a couple of years ago, he called me and said, "Jerry, I want to do something for you. I want to give you this building."

"Sir?" I said.

"I want to give you this building, and I want to give you the two lots that belong to the back of the building. But it all has to stay in the community."

I couldn't believe it. I went to discuss it with my family and with the association. A couple of weeks later, I was standing with Mr. Tudor in front of the building, and a man walked up and said he would give eighty thousand dollars for it. But Mr. Tudor replied, "I'm a man of my word, and I gave the building to this man right here."

So that's how we got our McElderry Park Community Association building and the land that provides the open greenspace that is part of Amazing Port Street.

My house is on that same street, and when I look out my back window, I can see the labyrinth. I've walked it a couple of times, but I prefer to just look at it. If things are getting on my nerves, I look at the labyrinth, and I feel calmer. I also feel proud. I think I appreciate it more because we made it, and I know it took hours and hours and hours. I look out, and I think, "We did that!" We still have crime in the neighborhood, but nothing like it was. I even heard one guy say to another, "Hey, man, you can't go back there."

It's a blessing from God what's happened here. I remember when we first started. I would tell people what we were going to do, and they would say, "You're going to do that here? Build that back there with all that crime?" But you've got to start somewhere. This was our start—and see how far we've gotten?

When in your stark and wintry despair,
you breathe the scent of springish air;
Search among the leaves of old
and find the offspring of the marigold.

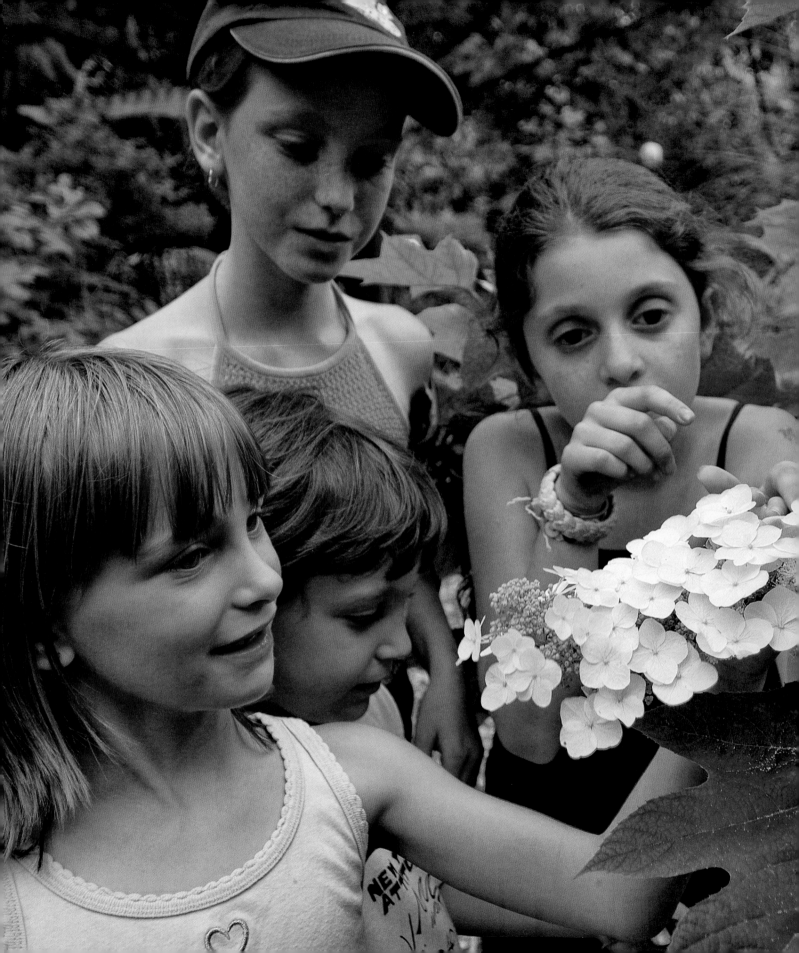

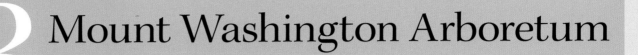

3 Mount Washington Arboretum

*So much can go wrong that you can
have no impact on. But in the garden,
you can create some beauty in a world
that is often ugly and disorderly.*

—Mike Sherlock, Firesoul

Tens of thousands of forgotten and unused urban lots dot the American landscape, attracting trash or worse. With dwindling municipal resources to turn these lots into community assets, most remain a detracting force. In Mount Washington, a neighborhood in northwestern Baltimore City, the citizens saw an abandoned lot and decided it could be something more. They decided that lot could become an arboretum.

The effort to turn that bleak urban land into a lush garden was led by Mike Sherlock, a pediatrician with a passion for horticulture. Mike saw this as an opportunity not only to beautify his neighborhood, but also to serve as a model of "what you can do in the city with abandoned lots that have humble soil."

Mike rallied his neighbors, raised funds, and took over that parcel overgrown with weeds and plagued by poor soil. He researched indigenous flora and fauna to create a garden that would thrive in its Mid-Atlantic climate and feed the native wildlife. He employed environmentally sound design elements, including an ingenious irrigation system that uses the stormwater runoff from a neighboring house to feed the soil.

What lessons do the butterflies have to teach? Where and when do their wings and spirits rest? Is transformation as easy as nature suggests? Beauty and grace is around and inside all the time. Goddess— help me be present.

A key element of the arboretum is its unique portal, which offers the chance to leave the frenzy of city life behind and step into the healing power of nature. Just feet from a busy, traffic-clogged street, the entry immediately transports visitors into a verdant forest. The rumble of cars is muted by the sounds of a gurgling waterfall and the wind through the leaves of the many trees that weren't there several years ago.

This arboretum is a reminder that the determination, imagination, and dedication to value the earth and to foster nature in a city are not limited to the creation of formal parks. This space wasn't planned by a planner; it wasn't an Olmsted-designed park. It came about, instead, from a private initiative, from a dedicated group of neighbors committed to change. A design process like this can be messy and imperfect, but it's honest. And it often results in a glorious space, such as this one. The neighbors put their souls into the arboretum, and the spirit of the natural setting is gratifying to the volunteers who maintain and care for it. The arboretum also provides a valuable retreat for the hundreds of visitors who now walk its paths. And perhaps one of those visitors will return to his or her own community, look at a vacant lot and think, "What if...?"

—T.S.

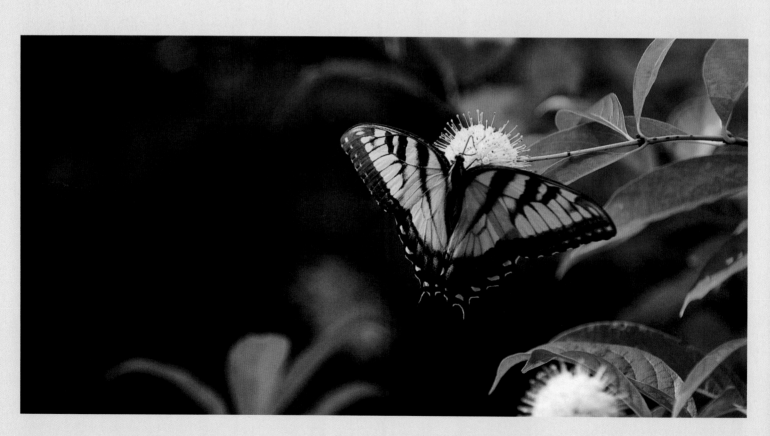

Mike Sherlock

Pediatrician

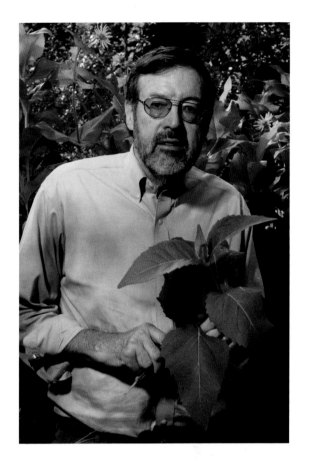

I grew up in Montana and spent most of my childhood playing outdoors. My mother spent a lot of time outdoors too. She was a fabulous gardener. She used to drag my brothers and me around her garden every day to look at her flowers. She'd say things like, "Boys, what do you think of my roses? Aren't they looking good?" And we'd answer, "Yes, Mom. Now can we go play?"

At some point, she ran out of space in our yard. She went to our neighbors on the right and asked if they'd mind if she "helped" with their backyard. "Oh no, Harriet," they said, "go right ahead." When that yard was full of flowers, she did the same thing with our neighbors on the left. The neighbors seemed to love it, but I was mortified to have my mother poking her nose—and her trowel—into other people's yards. It wasn't until I was in my thirties that I picked up a trowel. The irony is that once I started to garden, I became my mother, filling up every square inch of my yard.

At first, my motivation was purely practical. When I moved with my wife and family into our home in Mount Washington, I noticed that the plants there weren't doing so well, and I wanted to know why. I began researching, and after some time, I had a pretty good collection of garden books, along with healthier gardens in my yard. I enjoyed my research so much that I became certified in landscape design through George Washington University. Then I started a small landscaping business on the side with my sons, and we took care of a few gardens a year. In the meantime, I had planted my yard so full that there was no space left for anything more. Just like my mother, I said, "Now what?"

I began eyeing the public spaces in our neighborhood. At a major intersection, there was a traffic triangle planted with grass and crying out

Have reverence for all forms of life and they will take care of you.

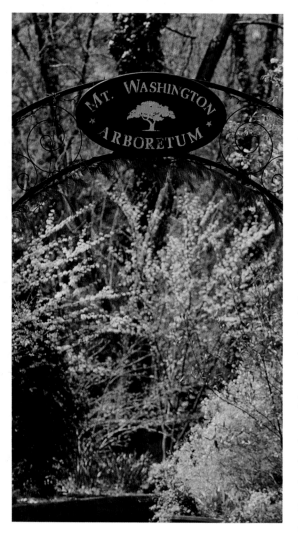

People travel around the world looking for a place like this. I'm happy that I only have to travel around the block!

for beautification. Unlike my shady yard, it got lots of sun, and I was eager to work with some different plants. I also thought that its central location made it the perfect place to plant a garden that our whole community could enjoy. So I called people in the neighborhood and raised about five hundred dollars for the project. Then I rounded up ten volunteers who liked to garden. After five or six hours of exhausting work, we had a lovely circular garden with black-eyed Susans and ornamental grasses.

The response from the neighborhood was very positive. Soon the Mount Washington Improvement Association asked me to start a committee to beautify other areas of the neighborhood, using its funding. Over the next ten years, our committee developed about twenty sites on public lands that ranged from bus stops to projects as long as 250 yards. We created a number of memorial gardens, one in memory of a community activist and another in memory of a beloved elementary school teacher. Eventually, we had land-scaped almost all the public spaces and were running out of places to work. It was then that we took a hard look at the most dismal acre of land in Mount Washington and embarked on our biggest project ever.

This acre had formerly been the site of a very nice garden apartment complex, with tennis courts and a swimming pool. In 1979, Hurricane David roared through the Mid-Atlantic, the nearby Western Run flooded, and the apartments were badly damaged. A year or two later, the City condemned the apartments, tore the buildings down, and claimed the land for the parks department. But nothing was ever done with the land, and it became over-grown. Then, the City and County put in a sewer line that went right through the middle of that area. They brought in heavy equipment and cleared it out until there wasn't a living thing left. The area was dug up and dynamited, and when the sewer line was laid, they filled up the holes and planted some trees. But most of the trees didn't survive, because the soil was so compacted by a year of heavy equipment driving over it.

The area had looked like a lunar landscape for about ten years, and we thought, "There has to be something better than this." But not everyone felt that we should take on a project of this magnitude. Some people thought that we had reached the limit of what we could take care of with our volunteer force. After weeks of discussion, the group decided to go ahead. We rolled up our sleeves and dug in—literally!

Every garden begins with the soil, and this soil was hard beyond what most gardeners can imagine. Picture a dirt parking lot; that's what we were working with. Not only was it so compacted that it was nearly impossible for plants to set down roots, it also had a lot of stones and debris from the

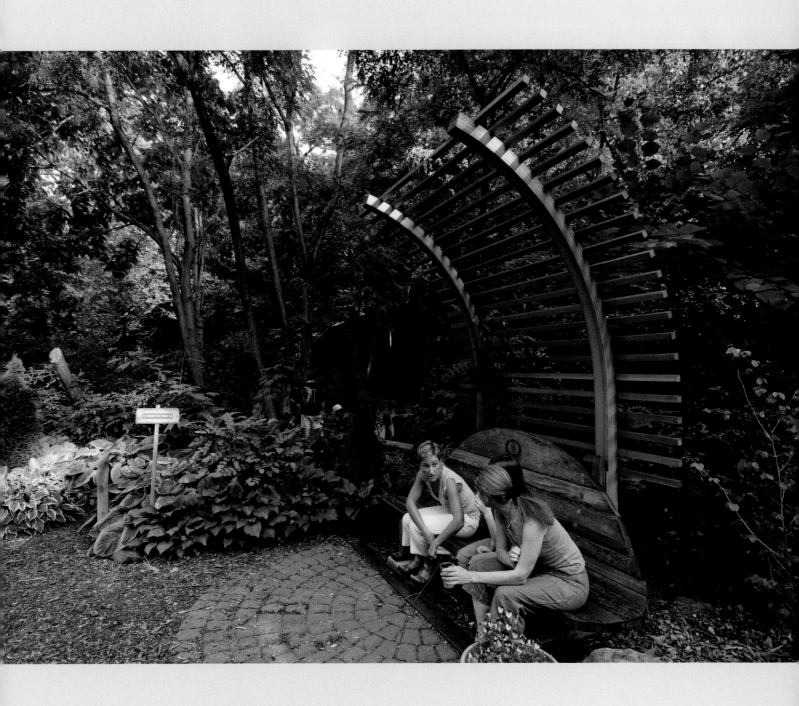

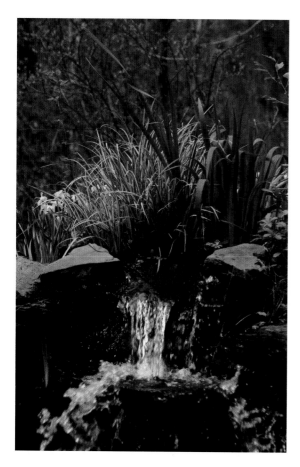

God sees us all as perfect and beautiful. We need to look at one another the same way. This is a perfect spot to reflect on His wonderful creation and love for us.

construction. So, with permission from the City, we created our own soil. Volunteers carried in hundreds of bags of mulch and laid down several inches of leaves. In a forest, it takes a hundred years to create an inch of topsoil; we had four to six inches of soil in just a few years. By doing this, we had created a blank canvas for planting—a prospect both exciting and daunting.

Our goal was to turn this acre into a habitat for native plants and animals. We wanted the space to welcome human visitors too, and instill in them an awareness of the value and beauty of native plants. Taking it one step further, we hoped to use the space to educate people to the value of habitat, even in a crowded city neighborhood. We wanted to use ecologically sound practices like composting, recycling garden wastes, and using green roofs and rain barrels, and we wanted to teach people how they could do the same thing in their own yards. Finally, we wanted our plantings to help prevent stormwater runoff from the site. We set the bar high for ourselves, but with thirty volunteers—a dozen committed to working an hour or so every Sunday—we've just about accomplished in seven years what we set out to do.

Today, we have more than three hundred species of trees, shrubs, and flowers growing in the arboretum, with 70 percent of them native to the Mid-Atlantic. "Native" means that they are useful to wildlife that lives here, such as birds, butterflies, and squirrels. In addition, we try to choose plants that have three-season interest. Our viburnum, for example, has flowers in the spring, which provide nectar for butterflies. Birds eat the plant's berries in the winter. In the fall, the leaves turn beautiful shades of yellow or orange. By contrast, azaleas and rhododendrons, while pretty when they bloom, are of little value to native wildlife because they haven't grown up together over the last ten thousand years: the birds and animals don't know what to do with these plants. The sweet gum is another of our best native trees. It has beautiful seeds on it in the fall, with little spikes on the pods that make it very ornamental. As soon as they ripen, the seeds drop to the ground, and the squirrels eat them.

The Native Americans who lived here for thousands of years knew very well that almost all plants have value in sustaining life. They might have had ten different uses for one plant—roots for one thing, the leaves to perhaps cure a toothache, the bark for something else. I have a particular interest in stories about how the Native Americans were connected to the land and used the plants, and knowing these stories makes me feel more connected with the plants we have here.

Over the years, we've created over three hundred yards of trails. The trails are curved, so that the park is not all revealed at once, but rather maintains a sense of mystery about what lies beyond the next turn. The arboretum has five benches, each placed in a different area so that visitors can enjoy the setting. One, of course, is the TKF bench with the journal. My son, David, who is a carpenter, added a curved arbor over the back of the bench. It is in an open circular area that invites groups to gather.

We have a 3,500-gallon pond with a waterfall, which serves as a centerpiece for fish, frogs, water bugs, birds, butterflies, and dragonflies. Water is always an issue for a gardener, and everything points to it becoming an even bigger concern as we consider the potential future effects of global warming. So David and I put our heads together and constructed a natural watering system to keep part of the arboretum sustainably irrigated. We created a contraption that pulls rainwater from the gutter of a nearby house, down a hill, and through an aqueduct that empties into a series of connected barrels. When one barrel fills, it overflows into the next. From there, the water flows into another aqueduct and empties like a waterfall into a water storage unit. When a half-inch of rain falls on that house up on the hill, we get about 600 gallons in our water storage unit, and hoses feed water to the field when needed. Our water containment area has a green roof, and we created a mini version of it so that we could show visitors how to build their own, using shale and hardy sedum.

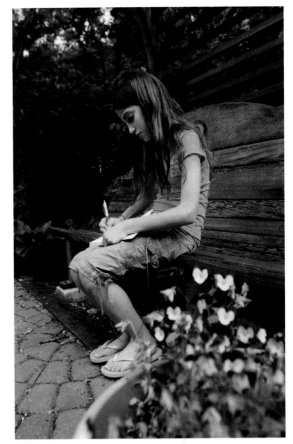

We use our teaching pavilion for all kinds of classes and programs open to the public, ranging from identifying plants to creating a native plant garden to controlling deer to making and using rain barrels. We recently held a symposium in the garden on water conservation and green roofs, and the garden writer from the *New York Times* introduced all the speakers. Many of the plants and trees are identified on plaques by both their common and botanical names, so the arboretum has become a field trip destination for Baltimore City schools. Kids and young adults come here to do community service. Painters and photographers use the natural setting for inspiration. Master gardeners and nature groups come here to learn. We're delighted at how much—and how respectfully—the arboretum is being used as a community resource.

It is also gratifying to see the variety of ways that people use this space. All day long, folks come and go. A woman sits by the pond almost every day to meditate. Mothers bring children; teenagers come by after school. Sometimes parents bring handicapped children here—our paths are wide enough and flat enough for wheelchairs. We've had people of different religions bring their holy books and sit and read. One day, I came down to do some work in the garden, and there was a man in formalwear sitting on the bench, meditating. I apologized for disturbing him. He told me that he was an Orthodox Jew, and

Gentle, peaceful breeze blows the cares away. Isn't it profound how nature can calm the spirit and refresh you? It is no wonder God created nature. His plan is in perfect balance.

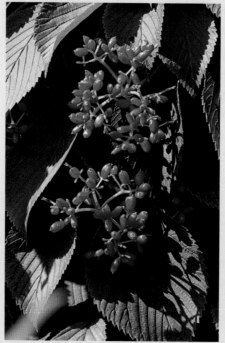

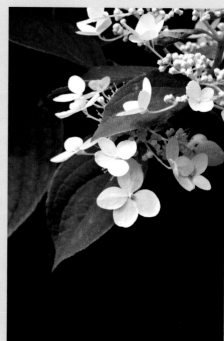

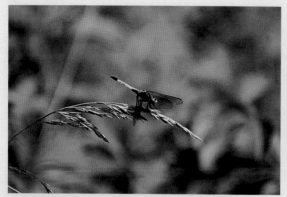

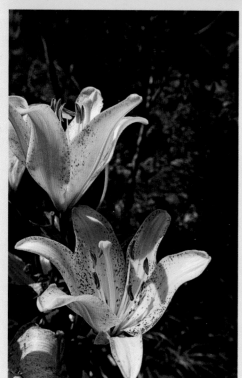

Someone is giving their time and love to maintain this lovely, sacred space. Why do you give this gift freely to me and other visitors? Thank you so much. This shows me that goodness can be—that many people are giving, kind, sharing, and love beauty.

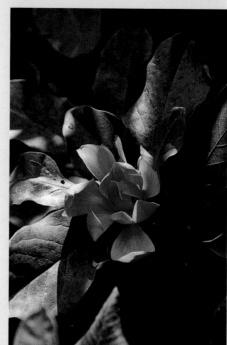

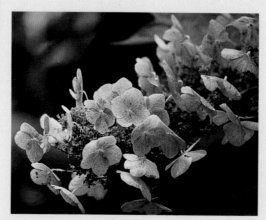

The spirit is here in our sacred place. It's name I cannot say, but we know.

he was preparing for his wedding in a couple of hours. Two couples, including my daughter and her husband, were married in this space. One summer afternoon, I walked into the circle, and there was a whole family asleep on the TKF bench—mother and father leaning against each other with their three small children sprawled across their laps! We hold summer and winter solstice celebrations and a Halloween party each year. On volunteer workdays, people in the community get to know each other while helping their neighborhood.

People often come up to me to thank me and tell me how much this garden means to them. One person in particular stands out in my mind—a woman visiting from Boston who told me she had lived in the apartments as a child. "What happened to this space was awful. To see my childhood home torn down, bulldozed, and devastated really hurt," she said. "But now it looks great. It feels like a wonderful rebirth of the place where I grew up."

I think that people love to come here because nature is so life-affirming. So often in the city, we lose sight of where we came from. In Europe, where I studied for one year, people spend more time outside—they spend time walking and being in their gardens. Here, we tend to lose touch. By building the arboretum, we have given ourselves and others a place to connect our busy lives with the natural rhythm of life. Most people pass through the other gardens we've created in Mount Washington, but here they stop and sit and stay. As a physician, I think that's good medicine!

There's another aspect of the garden—the spiritual aspect—that I must admit I was not fully aware of until people started pointing it out to me. My motivation for working on this arboretum was my fascination with plants. But from the very beginning, people have said things to me like, "I love it here. It's so spiritual." Hearing and reflecting on that has sparked something in me that goes beyond "Well, isn't that an interesting plant?" or "Isn't it neat how the Native Americans used it?" This garden, more than any other garden I've worked on, has made me aware of the spiritual dimension of gardening. And while I still spend most of my time in this garden working, not sitting, I feel as if I have more of a spiritual connection with nature than I had before doing the arboretum.

I hope—and I believe—that this acre of beauty that we've created has strengthened our community. There are about thirty volunteers who care for the arboretum. Some come every Sunday; others come three or four times a year to reconnect with each other. I see people walking in the garden that I know from the neighborhood, or adults that I knew back when they were children in Cub Scouts with my sons, or kids from the local school. I chat with them, and they chat with each other as they meet by happenstance in

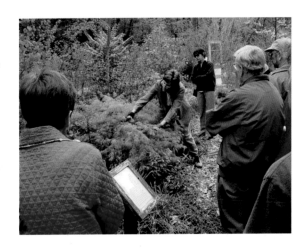

*Walk gently on this earth; don't harm even
    a leaf or blade of grass without
    thought.*
*Drive gently on our roads. Your car and
    your path are filled with beloved
    people and creatures.*
*Speak gently, each word can build a dream
    or break a heart.*
*Look gently on the whole creation, believing
    it is filled with the Divine, sometimes
    latent, sometimes in full glory, and
    all of it was created for your pleasure
    and benefit.*
*Enjoy life—to be happy at all times is a
    tremendous accomplishment,
    bringing you close to all mankind
    and creator, and your true self.*
*Live gently, cradling your own life, nurturing
    your own dreams, kissing your own
    sorrows, whispering soothing words
    to yourself.*
*Love gently, being sensitive to all you
    encounter, knowing all is connected.*
Rest gently...
    Sweet life, sweet dreams.

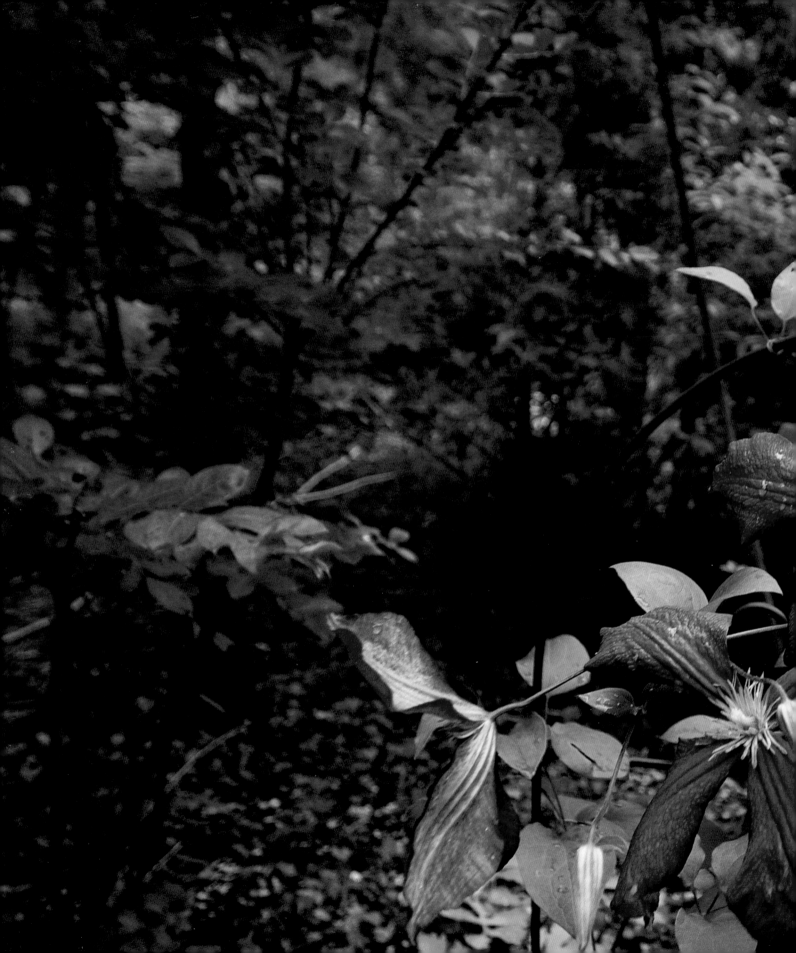

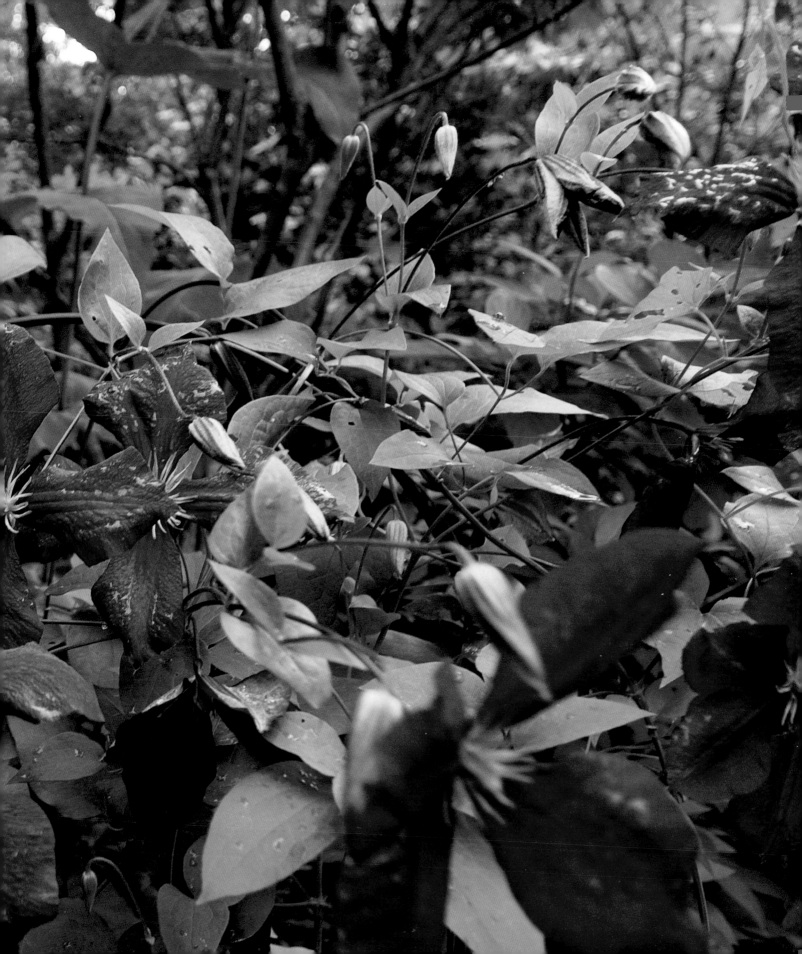

This place is a midday antidote to phones and hard drives, flickering fluorescent light and gray carpets that don't show dirt. I love the way the stems and branches lean out of their confined spaces, reaching every way at once. I love the way a flowering bush becomes a bouquet of butterflies and bees. I love how the boundary between earth and sky is not a straight line, marked instead by the individual curves of trees and leaves. I keep coming back for more.

the garden. All these little exchanges create a web of connectedness that makes our neighborhood a great place to live.

Just before I started on this project, my wife and I almost moved out of Mount Washington. It was my longtime dream to create an arboretum, and we had found a five-acre farm way out in the country that was perfect. It had a big hundred-year-old Amish barn with beautiful beams that we were going to restore. Then the whole deal fell through, and we were heartbroken. Shortly after that happened, this arboretum project began. Now I've put so much into it that I can't imagine ever leaving. It's like having a baby and then watching it grow up—you just don't walk away from that kind of joy.

I can understand perfectly now why my mother loved gardening and why she kept finding one space after the next to keep planting. So much can go wrong in this world that you can have no impact on. But in the garden, you

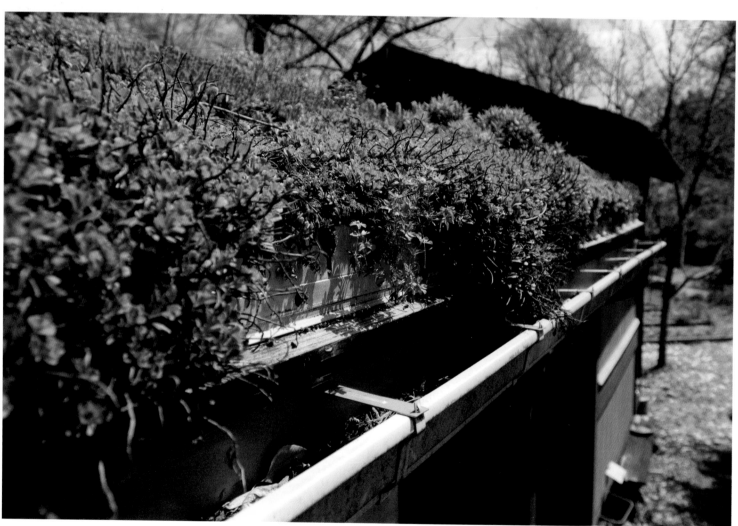

Green roof

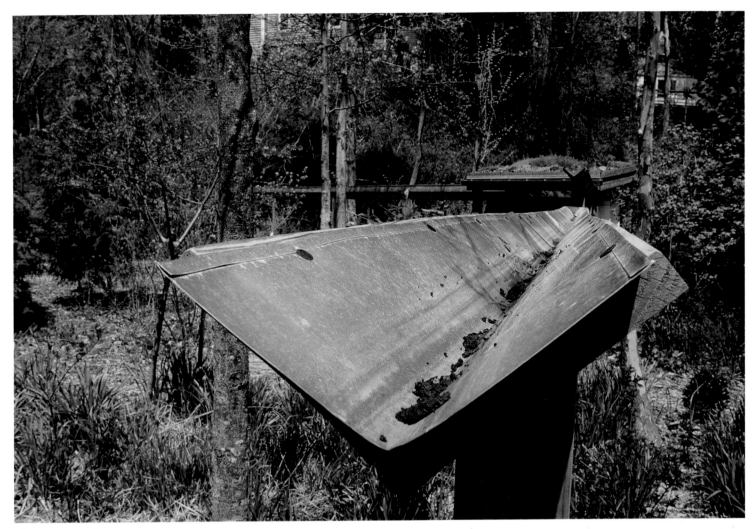

Rainwater aqueduct

can do something right. You can create some beauty in a world that is often ugly and disorderly. The garden puts you back in touch with the natural world and the natural order of things. A woman once stopped and asked me in a somewhat puzzled way if I was doing all this out of the goodness of my heart. I can't remember what I said to her, but later that day, the answer came to me. I, along with many others, am doing this for the good of my own heart. It's something I feel a deep need to do in a world that has grown increasingly materialistic and divorced from the natural world and from beauty in general. The arboretum is something I do because it fills my heart—and hopefully also the hearts of all those who come to visit.

Yom Kippur
—All places are sacred.
—All people are sacred.
—Today is a day to realize our inherent worth.
—Today is a day to recognize the beauty of our earth.
—Today is a day to look to the future and know that we can do good and be better.

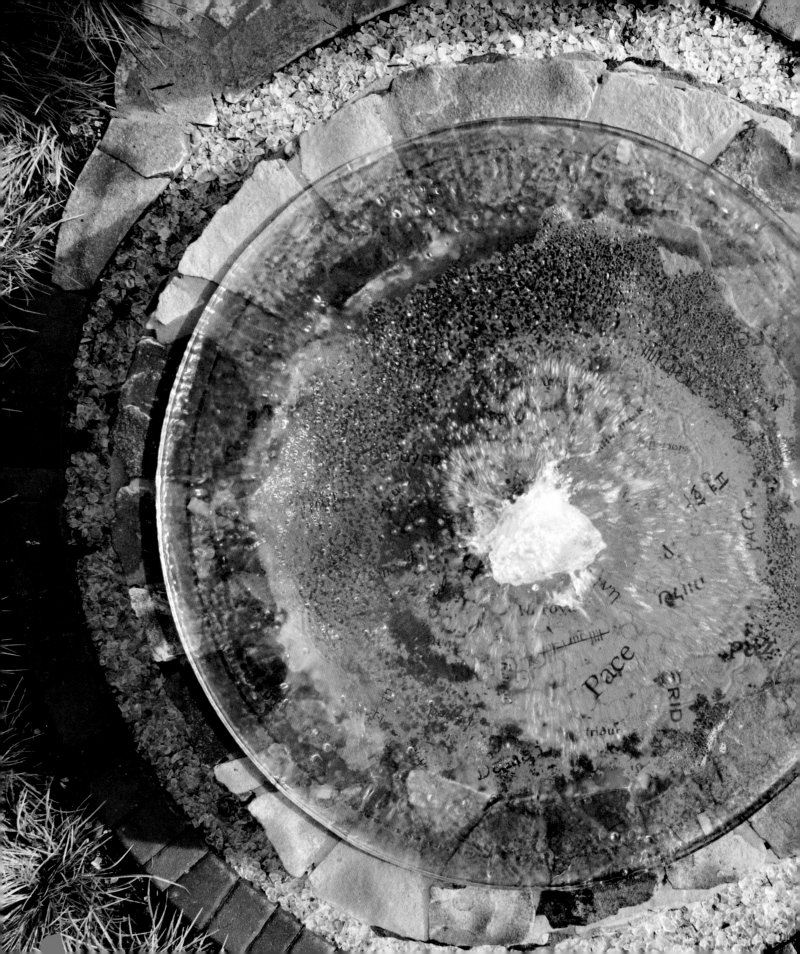

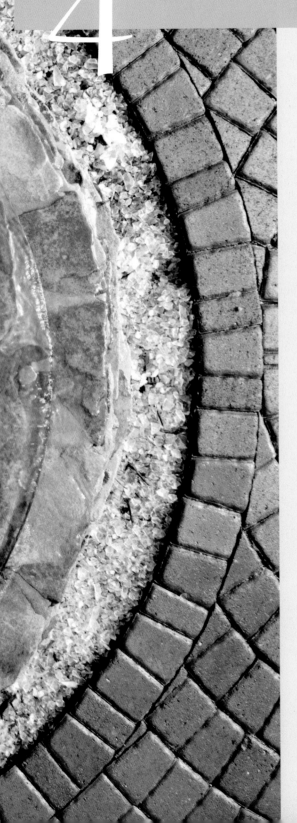

4 Garden of Peace and Remembrance

This garden experience has got me wanting to celebrate our universal hunger for peace and our universal hunger for remembering those who have gone before and influenced our lives.

— Father Tuck Grinnell, Firesoul

How do we move from a desire for tolerance to a true acceptance of others? The creation of an interfaith garden of peace and remembrance at St. Anthony of Padua Catholic Church inspired this provoking question. Located in Falls Church, Virginia, near Washington, D.C., St. Anthony sits in a very diverse community. The area is home to a growing number of new immigrants and a variety of languages and ethnicities. Father Tuck Grinnell has been the pastor at St. Anthony since 1994, and he found himself struggling with a disturbing reality. Many living in this community work hard just to make ends meet, and some families do not have enough money to bury their deceased.

Father Grinnell and his parish of 3,200 families dreamed of creating a columbarium, a place to inter ashes. They envisioned an open setting that could serve as a peaceful resting place not only for the church members, but also for the homeless, poor immigrants, and indigent in their community. The parish members hoped that in opening up the columbarium, they could

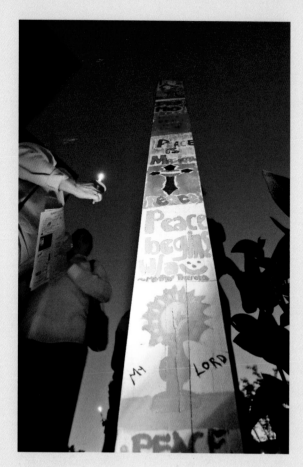

honor and remember the forgotten and those from distant lands dwelling among them.

In addition to the columbarium, they wanted to create a garden for reflection and respite. The challenge for the parish was to take an enclosed space that was surrounded on three sides by the church and rectory, and make it feel accessible to the entire community. Father Tuck enlisted the help of pastoral counselor Pauline Flynn, architect Mario Pareja, and master gardener and landscape designer Dorothy Schmitt to help realize the design and to draw upon the resources and energy of the whole of Falls Church. But creating a truly open space was not an easy prospect. It meant opening up their own parish to a very broad community. It meant getting outside of their comfort zone. The team members grappled with developing a multifaceted, inclusive approach, and they ultimately took the courageous step of inviting intercultural and interfaith groups to be part of the visioning process.

The collaborative effort resulted in the aptly named Garden of Peace and Remembrance. The garden's path leads visitors through a forest of peace poles, each one eight feet high and distinctively decorated. As visitors stroll down the stone walkway toward the bubbling peace fountain, the lush garden embraces them with its splendor of textures, colors, and fragrances. Beyond the fountain, a columbarium holds in repose the ashes of the deceased. Throughout the garden, benches beckon to people to sit in the midst of this beauty. The garden is open to all and is truly a place of respite for those in need of comfort or simply a moment of silence in the midst of a bustling and highly diverse community. The space serves both as a gathering spot for the broader community and as a location for quiet meditation. In this garden, nature serves to unify a diverse populace and to remind those who enter that we are all equal, that we are all in it together.

—T.S.

This is a place of peace for every faith as long as you are with God (whatever you call him) because God is good and you can feel it in this garden. Thank you, St. Anthony, for giving an opening from heaven. I come here and I am not Catholic, but I feel it is ok. Thank you again.

Father Tuck Grinnell

Pastor, St. Anthony of Padua Catholic Church

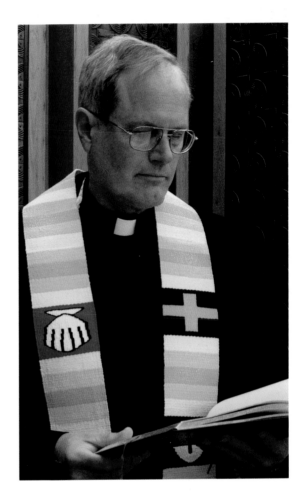

As a pastor in a very diverse community, I have ministered to dying people who have no place to inter their ashes. There are many people who work hard all their lives but never at the kind of job that offers a retirement fund. When they get to old age, they're living on vapors. They may be on Medicaid, but when they die, there is nothing left—and the cost of burial is stunning. Even the cost of placing ashes in a columbarium can be as much as three thousand dollars, which might as well be a million dollars for some people. These people deserve a final resting place, and families want a physical place where they can come to remember their loved ones.

For a long time, I had dreamed of having a columbarium at the church with space reserved for all God's children—niches for people who can pay to have their ashes placed there, and niches reserved for people who can't afford to pay. In fact, I thought the empty space outside my office window would be a perfect place for a garden with a columbarium. It was a square of grass, surrounded by the high walls of the church and buildings that we use for pastoral counseling and offices. Otherwise, there was nothing there. I envisioned a space that could be both beautiful and useful, but we didn't have the money to create that. In fact, it was such an impossible dream that I had put it in my file titled "When someone dies and leaves me a million dollars..."

When the TKF Foundation became interested in our project, we really began to imagine what could be—and we had to think much bigger than we had up to that point. Our original plan for a garden included Christian statuary and other denominational symbols, but to qualify for support, we had to create an "open" garden. Not only open to anyone and everyone beyond our parish, but also open in the sense that it would have no icons, statues, or symbols except ones that are open to and understood by all. That really got me thinking and was one of the most exciting aspects of the project for me. What would that look like—a garden that had universal appeal and was welcoming to everyone? What would our garden express?

The Peace Garden is the most welcoming, compelling, and relevant place on earth. Those who created this precious outdoor sanctuary have brought us all closer to God.

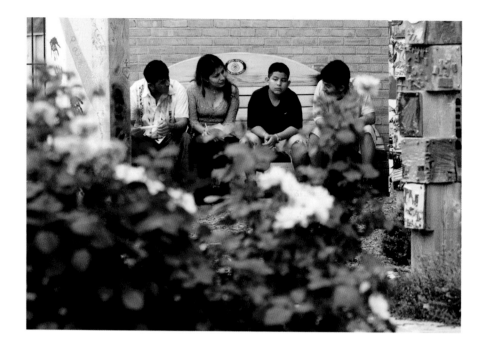

Es una ofrenda a Dios hermosa sin color y sin discriminación a ninguna raza aquí todas ante Dios somos sus hijos.

Always a quiet and restful place, no matter what is happening around and inside me. Peace is in the air here. I breathe it in when I am here, and I can smell it in the wood of the bench.

Thank you, kind hands who crafted and placed this bench. Thank you, Deep Mystery, for bubbling into our lives.

It was our good fortune to have extremely talented and creative people working on this. Mario Pareja is an architect in our parish, and he designed the garden pro bono. Dorothy Schmitt is a master gardener, and her knowledge and donation of countless hours have given our garden its perfect sense of balance. Her son, John, put in all the hardscape at cost; he was putting the finishing touches on it right up to the night before the dedication of the garden. Pauline Flynn had the daunting task of pulling together all the meetings and coordinating the project.

Many serendipitous things happened to move the project along. For example, when we were grappling with the question of how to draw people into the garden, I happened to participate in the dedication of a chapel in a local hospital. One of the imams from a nearby mosque was also there. I was talking about the peace garden, and he mentioned in an offhand manner, "My wife did a peace pole." I had never heard of a peace pole, so he described it to me. I took the idea back to the committee, and that grew into the forest of peace poles through which visitors enter our garden. I love the way the gift of that idea was delivered.

So now, instead of a lifeless, useless patch of grass, we have a beautiful Garden of Peace and Remembrance. Helping to create it has been a terrific experience for me and has changed me in several important ways. First of all, as I've gotten older, I've grown to love God's nature more and more. So I love that I was involved in a project to create greenspace. I love the roses and the trees. I love the red bark of the Japanese maple in winter. I love the texture of the stone in the fountain and on the walkways.

Second, thinking about how to put something together that would have universal appeal and universal significance has expanded my thinking. My job is to convince people to embrace the Christian faith and the Church—that's what I do and what I like to do. But this garden experience has got me wanting to celebrate our universal hunger for peace and our universal hunger for remembering those who have gone before and influenced our lives. The columbarium will feed that hunger. If you're a child of God who dies with enough, you have a place. And if you're a child of God who dies without enough, you still have a place.

Third, the process of creating this garden was challenging on an interpersonal level. It was painful for all of us—Mario, Dorothy, Pauline, and myself—to give up our individual visions for the garden. I think that I was able to defuse some difficult moments not by authority but by enthusiasm, and I'm sure, now that the garden is complete, we all feel that what we created together far surpasses anything we could have done individually. I think the TKF vision of what gardens can do for the human spirit is exactly what the postmodern world needs. People feel deeply fragmented and yet open to a spiritual awakening that is almost preconscious. A garden is exactly the environment people need to open the door to mystery and spirituality.

Finally—and this is a delightful discovery for me—I think I have a bit of artist in me. I've never considered myself an artistic person—maybe with

You can't walk through the gates of the Peace Garden without the feeling of serenity . . . It slows you from the fast pace of the northern Virginia lifestyle. It's a great addition to this area. St. Anthony of Padua would be proud to see a place of peace like this.

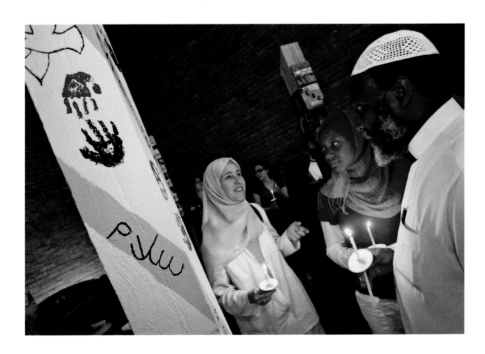

words but certainly not with design or concepts or materials or plants. But having the good fortune to work with architects and gardeners and other artists has sparked something in me. Now when I'm out and about and see blank spaces, I envision how they could be transformed into something that has multiple layers of meaning. I can think outside the box in a way I never could before, and it carries over to all parts of my life.

For me, the final piece of this project is to increase the use of the garden. We have prayers for peace in the garden once a month, and every September we have an interfaith prayer service on the International Day of Peace. People walk in the garden. I look out and see them sitting on the benches, reading, or meditating. School children sometimes come to this quiet place for writing assignments. One of our pastoral counselors has her clients, especially couples, spend time in the peace garden after a session. But I can envision so much more, and I know that over time this garden of peace and remembrance will bear a lot more fruit. It will because of all the prayers for peace that are sent out from it.

Dear God, please end war forever! I don't like people going against each other. It is horrible! You made us to be friendly to each other, not to go against each other. I love peace and quiet.

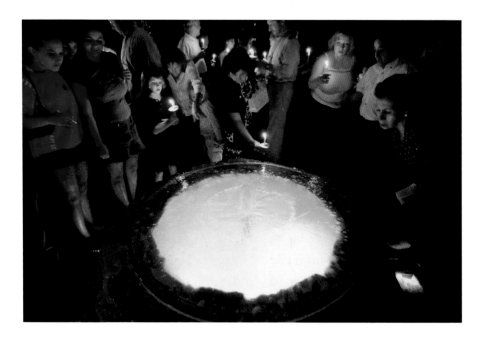

Mario Pareja

Architect

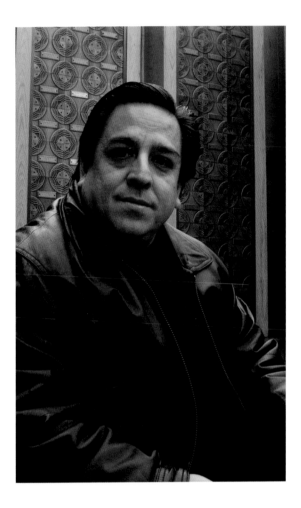

The architectural challenge was to take what's called a *negative space* and turn it into a garden that would be a vibrant, living part of our community, a welcoming space whose symbols could be understood by anyone who walked in. Our committee worked for months to decide what those symbols would be, and it was my job to turn them into a garden design.

We agreed that the circle would be the primary element of the design, because it is a symbol of inclusiveness. The circle exists in civilizations throughout the world and is a focal point for gathering, and we wanted our garden to be a gathering place for our whole community. People enter the garden on a curved stone walkway that leads them to a circular stone courtyard where there is a fountain.

We chose water to represent peace. Flowing water, like our hunger for peace, is constant. No matter how many times we are knocked down in our quest for peace, it is important that we get up and keep on trying, just as rivers keep flowing. Our fountain is a representation of this concept. It is made of rough-cut fieldstone, representing the earth, hardship, and the rough edges of humanity. Rather than tilting outward or being cylindrical, the fountain is shaped like a beehive, which naturally draws people in toward it. By that gesture of leaning in, people become part of the peace fountain, rather than just spectators.

When they lean in, they see that on top of the stone base is a glass plate on which the word *peace* is engraved in eighty languages, each language representing one of the cultures in our parish and community. But once we decided to use that word, we had to decide how to order the different languages. Alphabetically? Geographically? How could we put them in order without giving one more importance than another? Then another dedicated

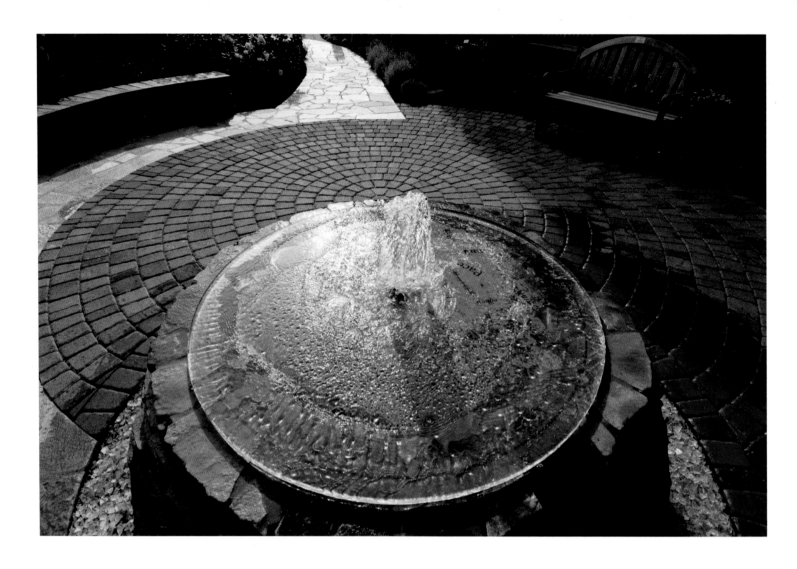

The water alone is a soul soother!
The sound of the water gentles me.

member of the design committee had a great idea. She picked up our eighty pieces of paper, each with *peace* written in a different language, and she threw them in the air. Where they fell became the design we used on the glass plate.

We considered using a granite plate, because glass is fragile and can break. But for that very reason—because peace is also fragile and can be easily broken—we chose glass. Water flows over the top of the glass and down the stone sides of the fountain into a pool, signifying that when peace is flowing into and out of our hearts, it can overcome any obstacle, just as water, over time, will smooth the roughness of the stone. The fountain sits a little off-center in the garden, and there is a reason for that. When people walk to the fountain, they themselves are actually closer to the center of the garden, symbolizing that humans are the central force in creating peace. In the well around the bottom of the fountain, there are hundreds of glass pieces representing the tears shed in heartbreak for all the times humans have been at odds or at war with each other, rather than at peace.

To the right of the peace fountain stand two beautiful large, upright stones known as *steles*. They face north, and they are symbols of one of the few things that humanity agrees on absolutely—the direction north. They represent a starting place for peace. Beside the steles are two benches shaped to follow the curve of the circle. The bases are fieldstone; one is topped with wood, the other stone. The wood is smoother and more comfortable to sit on. The stone is harder, representing the hardships that humanity seems destined to endure. I find it interesting to watch which bench people choose to sit on. I think it is probably tied to their psyche. Younger people tend to sit on the stone, while older people prefer the smoother wooden bench, perhaps because they have experienced life's roughness and are ready for some smooth sailing.

Speaking of smooth sailing, there were times on the committee when it wasn't. For example, there is one curved path that leads people from the entrance of the garden to the fountain. My original proposal was to have two paths, because I think that life is made up of many roads, and all of us don't necessarily take the same road to get to a destination. That idea was important to me, but the committee rejected it because they thought there wasn't enough space. That was hard for me to accept. But it was part of the process and presented me with one of the most important lessons of this project—to listen better and to accept leadership from others. Sometimes as an architect,

Gracias Dios por este hermoso y tranquilo jardín donde se siente la paz Divina y la unión de todos nuestros hermanos en Jesús.

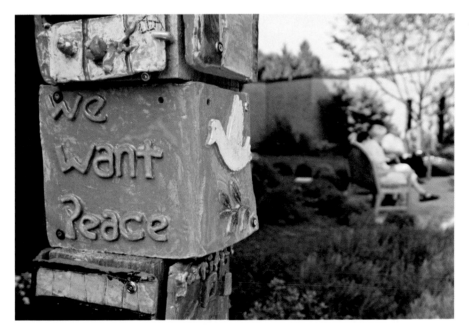

I am sitting in this sacred space thinking of all good people who have lived, are living, and will someday live.

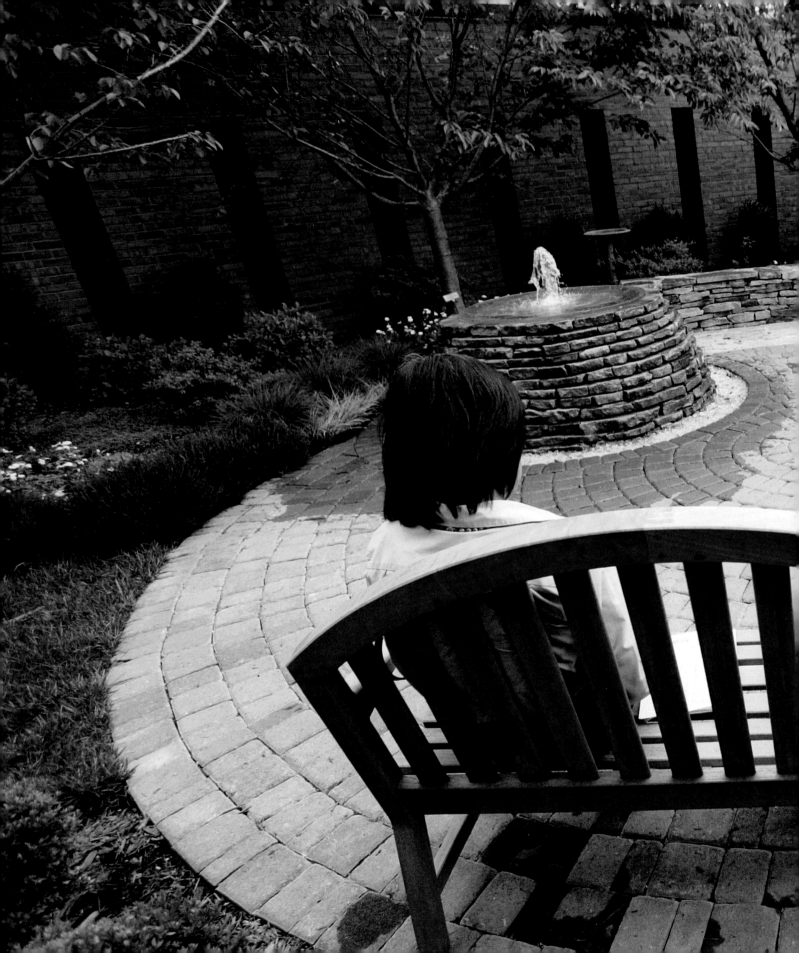

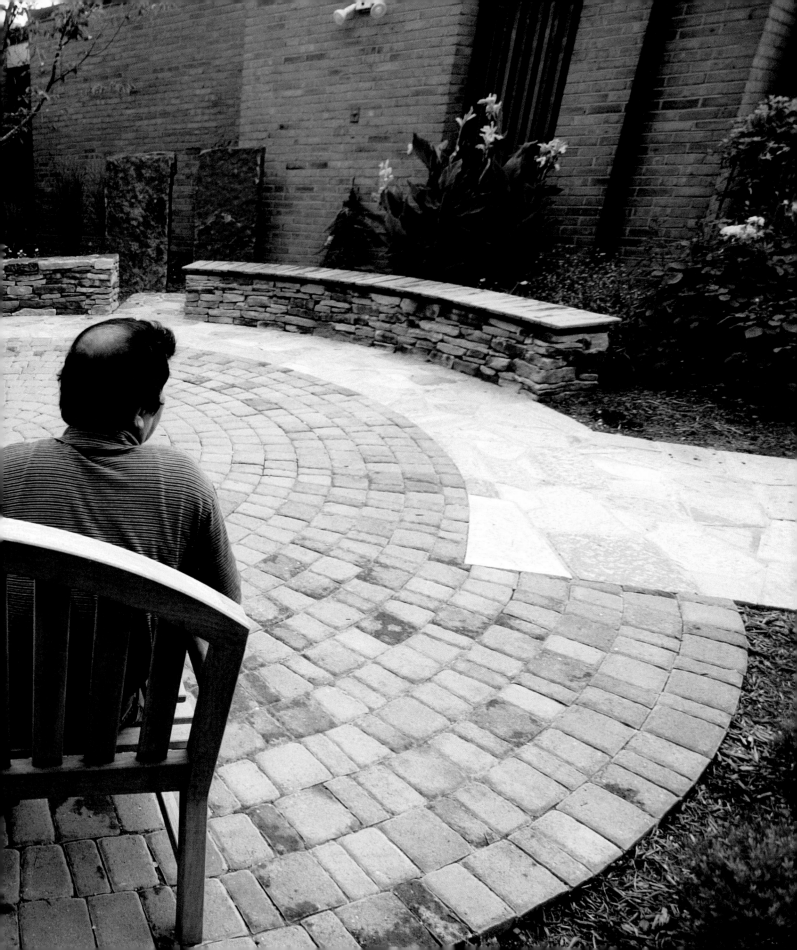

The ache in my heart from the recent death of my father was soothed by the beauty and calm in this garden. We were so privileged to have him all these years. Thank you, God, for blessing us with life and sharing him with us.

you can *not* listen to people. You can take the attitude that your way is the right way and plow on through. With this project, that was not possible. To have peace, you have to work together, whether you're trying to create a garden or a world where people get along. All of us on the committee learned to work together toward one goal, and in the end, I felt spiritually much closer to people I hadn't known before. That's a lot to be grateful for.

The way I satisfied both the committee and myself was to use stones of various textures in the path, so that visitors have the subtle feeling that there are different paths there. As visitors enter through the peace poles, they get the feeling of being in a forest—as in the well-known poem "The Road Not Taken." The eleven peace poles were designed by groups from St. Anthony's, from neighboring faith communities, and from public and private schools. If a visitor stands on the brass marker embedded in the walkway, he or she becomes a symbolic wandering twelfth peace pole, taking peace out into the world.

Tucked in the back of the garden is the columbarium for the reposal of ashes, which I think is quite beautiful. I created five vertical niches on the church wall, and while people probably aren't aware of it, each is about the size of an upright coffin. Each is finished in cypress, a very hard wood that has been used in many cultures and religions throughout time for the burial of important people. The area surrounding the "coffins" is finished with copper, again a symbolic choice. Copper is a metal that doesn't stay one color but is constantly changing and aging through time. That change keeps this area alive and dynamic.

As an architect, you can never really know how people will react to the architectural elements around them. I doubt that most of the people who come here think about all the symbolism in this garden on a conscious level. But I have no doubt that they experience peace, because I've been told so by many people. Often, they simply say, "There's something about this garden; it feels so good." Like peace, if we can achieve it.

Pauline Flynn

Pastoral Counselor and Project Manager

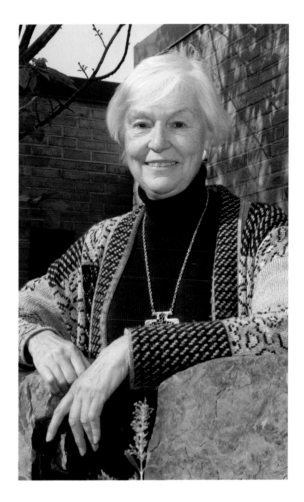

At the time the Garden of Peace and Remembrance was created, I was a pastoral counselor at St. Anthony's. As I see it, the ultimate goal of any pastoral counselor is to help people discover, or rediscover, their dream for themselves. And what I have learned as a pastoral counselor and therapist is that the deepest dream of every human heart is peace, inner peace.

Our garden began with a dream: Father Tuck's vision for a garden. This was very exciting for me because as part of my work for the pastoral counseling program, I had designed a presentation on backyard spirituality and had created a sacred space in my own backyard. Now I had an opportunity to help create a much larger sacred space. TKF challenged us to be as inclusive as possible, so we began by holding two charrettes—meetings designed to bring people together to discuss possibilities. Because I was passionate about the idea, I offered to organize these meetings, by identifying all the neighborhood groups, schools, churches, faith communities, and businesses and inviting them to participate. It was a major task, but it was absolutely worth the effort.

When the design committee decided that peace poles would be part of the garden, I took on the job of finding groups to design the peace poles. Again I contacted the neighboring faith groups and public and private schools, with the result that our forest of peace poles was created by five public schools, two private religious schools, three religious communities in our area, a youth group, and one individual. In the case of the public schools, middle- and high-school students mentored the elementary students, helping to guide the creation of their poles. The guidelines we gave them were very simple—they could use whatever images they thought of that related to peace, but we encouraged them to use symbols and languages that came from their own cultures. We are forever grateful to the teachers who inspired and supervised the students as they put their hearts into these magnificent poles.

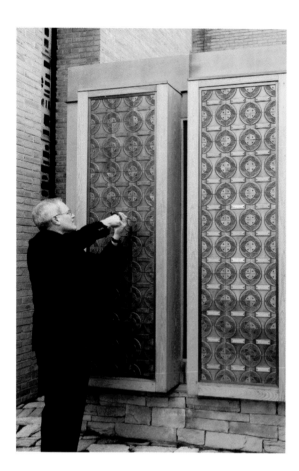

Gracias a Dios por el milagro del Jardín de Paz donde puedo hablar con mi hijo.

The local public elementary school has students from seventy-three countries; forty-two different languages are spoken there. The children designed their pole in a tile medium using a mosaic of colors that are representative of the rich cultural diversity of the school. The local Episcopal church, almost 150 years old, has seen a lot of changes in the community. Its pole welcomes visitors by declaring the ancient street greeting in the two predominant languages of our community: "Peace be with you" and "La paz sea con ustedes."

I think it's fascinating that the children of the school at St. Anthony's and the children at the community Islamic school created poles that are very similar, both using the handprints of the children. For the Islamic children, whose families come from nineteen different countries and have experienced both good and bad times, the hands represent people from all around the world reaching out to each other to spread peace. The children of St. Anthony's, after discussing the meaning of peace, studying the work of a famous artist, and brainstorming, used their handprints to transform the wooden pole into a charming patchwork quilt, which is peaceful and calming.

The peace pole that draws the most attention is the one created by our local middle school. The school building was being rebuilt at the time of this project. With art supplies in the process of being moved, the students had to make do with what they could find. What they found was telephone wire and plastic bullet boxes! The empty boxes were given to them by the police officer assigned to the school. When the children found out what the boxes were, they didn't think they were appropriate for a peace pole. But then they realized that if they attached the boxes to the peace pole backward, no one could ever put another bullet into them. They thought that made a powerful statement about peace, and so they decorated the entire pole with reversed bullet boxes. Together, the eleven poles create a joyful celebration of the many cultures that make their home in our community.

The plantings in the garden—their colors, scents, and textures—play a major role in creating the feeling of peace that people experience in this space. The trees were carefully chosen by Dorothy Schmitt and planted by her son, John. Dorothy chose three Yoshino cherry trees, which are round and full and nearly conceal the rectory wall behind them. Against the high walls of the church, she planted three English hornbeams, trees that grow vertically in a shape that suggests praying hands. The marvelous thing about the plantings and the architecture of this garden is that it all creates the feeling of being held in a closed space, safe and at peace. And yet the garden is completely open in the sense of being open to all.

I have to say that when I was working on the garden, I really did not understand for a long time what TKF meant by *open*. I was focused on the *sacred*. Now I have come to the conclusion that the garden is more *sacred* because it is so *open*. Everything in the garden—the water, the fountain, the plants and trees and stones, the pathways, the word *peace* in eighty languages—speaks directly to each visitor. Our garden is open because every symbol is universally understood. Even though it is in the courtyard of a Catholic church, there are no barriers that exclude people from other faiths or ethnic groups. I believe this symbolic unity of people is what creates the feeling of deep peace that visitors feel when they come into this space.

Our goal was to create a place that is a living tribute to our yearning for peace, a place where people can find peace within themselves and then take it out into the community. I believe we succeeded in doing that. There is a spot in the garden where one can stand, looking out toward the gate, and see the peace pole with these words: "Go in peace" and "Vayan en pax." For me, that says it all.

帝全平
上安和

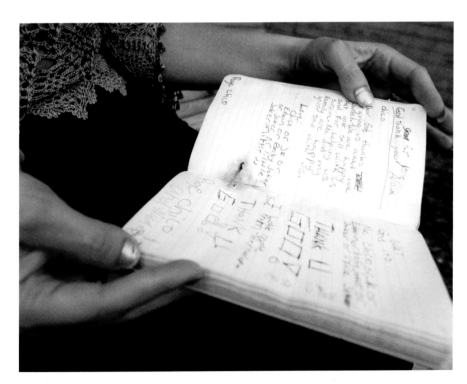

This book transcends us beyond here and now, proving we can be universally whole when at peace.

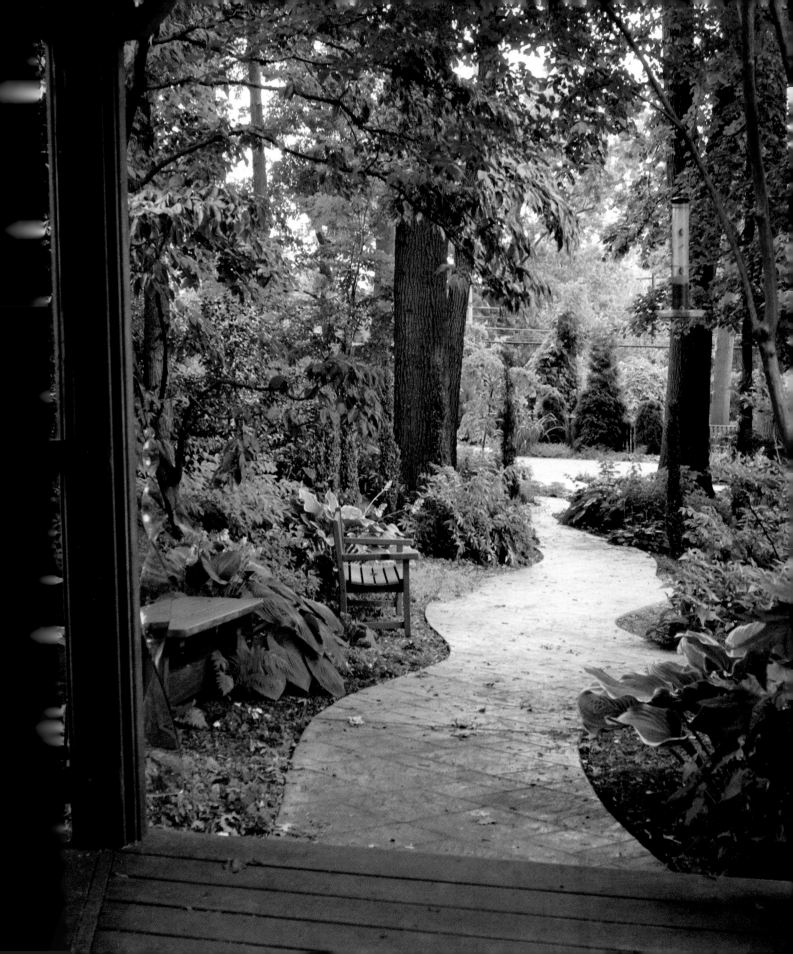

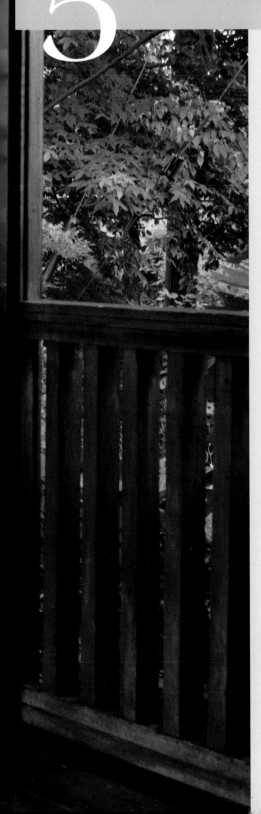

5 Whitman-Walker Healing Garden

The theme of loss is universal—as is the desire to be healed and whole.

—Geof Lindstrom, Firesoul

Affecting millions of people around the world, HIV/AIDS is one of the greatest epidemics of our time. It has brought with it a stigma that has spread as fast as the infectious disease itself, isolating the very people who need help and support the most.

In the mid-1990s, at a time when people were still nervous to be around those infected with HIV, the Whitman-Walker Clinic of Northern Virginia moved to a new location. The new building looked out onto a sizeable area of overgrown woodland covered with brambles and trash. In its stead, the clinic staff members envisioned a beautiful space, a sheltering place for patients struggling with a new reality—a healing garden.

This healing garden emerged under the guiding hand of designer Geof Lindstrom. A force of volunteers, including sculptor Caroline Hufford-Anderson, whose own son had died of AIDS, joined Geof. Together they created a labyrinth, with a meditative path that offers patients the opportunity to gain perspective in the midst of great physical and emotional change. Honoring the needs of its primary users, the clinic placed artistic and architectural features significant to the patients throughout the labyrinth. They enlisted Karen Rowe to maintain the labyrinth and to coordinate activities around the site.

At first, this garden was closed—designed to remove everyone affected by the disease, including patients' family and friends, to a secure place away from the community, where they could turn to each other for comfort. But with continued medical research, improved treatment, and time, the patients' quality of life began to improve. As a result of this newfound confidence, the clinic decided to fully open this sacred space to the surrounding communities. The decision has brought critical added support, and perhaps just as important, a newfound acceptance of those with HIV/AIDS. Today, this garden is utilized by the entire neighborhood and is helping to usher in a new era for those with HIV/AIDS.

—*T.S.*

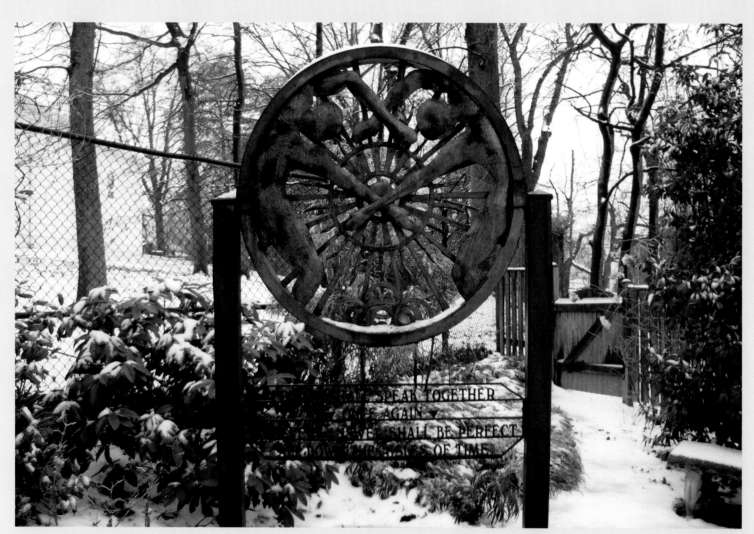

Promise by Caroline Hufford-Anderson

Caroline Hufford-Anderson

Sculptor and Healing Garden Volunteer

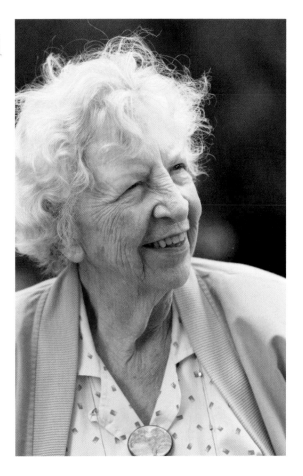

Several years ago, my son Henry, a young lawyer in Tucson, called me. "Mother, please sit down," he said. "This is the hardest call I've ever made, but I have something to tell you."

"What? What?" I asked, frightened.

"I have something called HIV," he said, "and it probably will develop into AIDS."

His statement hit me like a thunderbolt. I knew very little about AIDS—just enough to fear it. Henry also told me that he was gay, a fact I had never known, nor had I even surmised. We talked for some time. Henry tried to reassure me that he had a long time left to live.

When the call ended, I could scarcely walk. After my senses returned, I knew that I had to learn all I could about AIDS, how I could help my dear son. I went to the Whitman-Walker Clinic in the District of Columbia and talked with a caseworker.

I made many visits to Tucson, and my relationship with Henry deepened. I was with him on the day he died, five years later. One thing became clear, pointed out to me by Henry himself. "I'm the same son you've always known, Mother," he said. "The same. I just understand myself better."

This experience with my son brought me a new comprehension of the range of God's marvelous creation. How reasonable and logical that in the infinite complexity of God's art, human sexuality, like every snowflake, should take on its own individual pattern and shape. How precious is each work made by God's hand!

I'm thankful for the lifting of that veil from my eyes, and I'm grateful to have been involved in creating a space that could serve as a bridge to the community—so that others, like myself, might grasp new understandings.

Three times around the labyrinth—once for how far I have already come, twice for where I am now , and thrice for where I am yet to go.

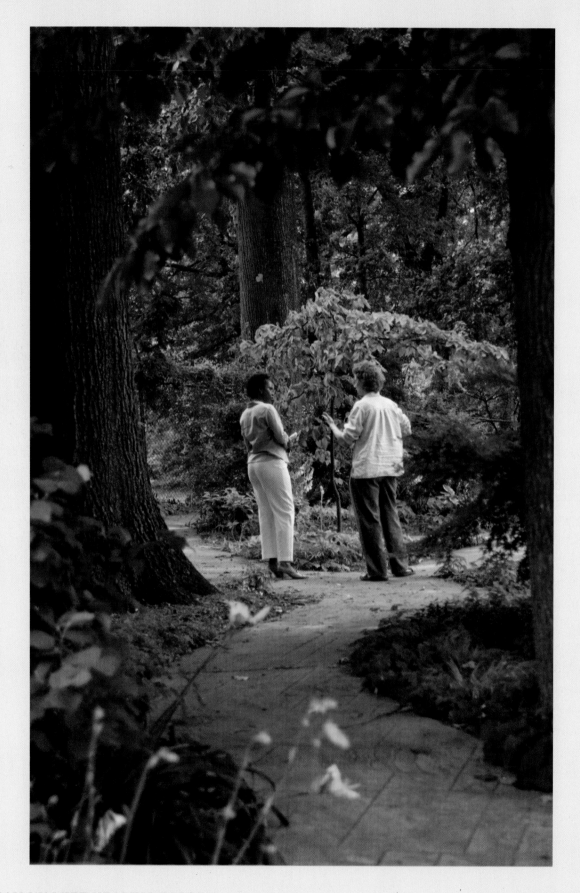

Geof Lindstrom

Landscape Designer and Gardener

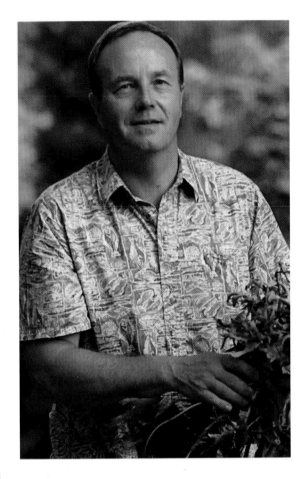

I've never been a big joiner, but when the organizer of the healing garden at the Whitman-Walker Clinic approached me, it felt really important that I get involved.

The clinic was in a cinderblock building that used to house a local radio station. At the time, there was nothing behind it but weeds and trash and cement slabs. Inside, there were tiny little waiting rooms with people sitting cheek to jowl with one another, miserable and scared. This was before the medicines available today that enable HIV/AIDS patients to live longer, healthier lives. Illness and death were all around. There was practically no one in the gay community who hadn't been to a clinic like this—either to obtain care for himself or to sit with a friend. It was grim. The clinic was on a shoestring budget, and there were no resources to try to make the experience better for people—at just the moment when a softer, nicer environment would have meant so much.

The vision of Jay Fisette, director of the clinic, and the primary goal of the healing garden committee, was to create a place of hope and encouragement for those living with the disease and those who love them. I've spent the latter part of my life creating gardens for people, and I thought, "What could be better than to help by doing something I love?" So I joined the effort, and for me, it was a surprising and wonderful introduction to the joys of volunteer work. It's a good thing I liked it so much, because within about a year, the original designer and organizer, Drew Fitzmorris, moved away, and I and all the other members of the committee found ourselves with a lot of work to do!

The other goal of the garden was to build a bridge between the clinic and the community. At the time the garden was conceived in the mid-1990s, people were still nervous about being around anybody with AIDS or being associ-

So much having to let go, let go. Hope I'll not have to let go of this sacred space too. True, all space is sacred, if we only knew, but we need places of retreat and special beauty like this to help us awaken to the sacred everywhere.

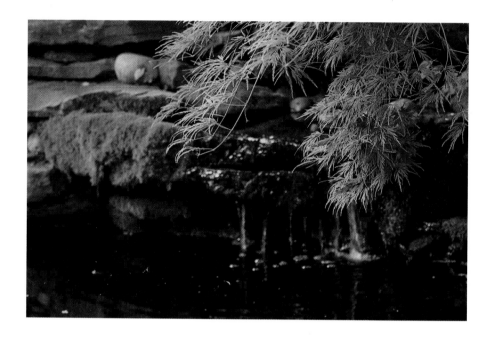

This is a place where spirits meet—
those who are living in this earth
and those who are living in the next.
May we learn of love from the kindred who
have gone beyond our limited vision.
May we learn our lessons well.

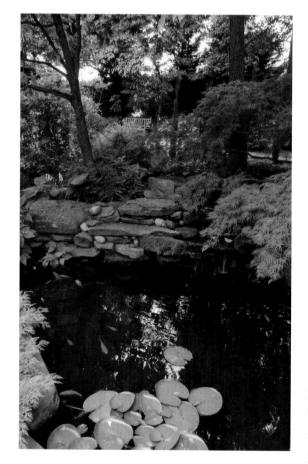

ated with anything that had to do with AIDS. There were a lot of walls then: walls of secrecy around the people with HIV/AIDS that kept them isolated and walls that people in the community put up to keep themselves separated. We hoped to break down some of those walls by creating a place of beauty and peace that would be open to the community and that would encourage people to come to the clinic grounds, use the lovely space, and, hopefully, learn more about the illness.

I'm a confirmed believer in serendipity. If something is meant to happen, things will fall into place. If not, they won't. Everything fell into place for the healing garden, so I have to think the time was right for it. I joined the project when it was in its infancy. While the committee had enthusiasm and a plan, it had no money. At the time, I was also on the board of a nonprofit foundation whose goal was to foster a higher quality of life for gays and lesbians. I helped secure a small grant for the clinic that enabled us to take our first step forward by putting in a patio and seating wall in the area we had cleared. Even more importantly, this action demonstrated that the healing garden was a serious effort. Before long, with the fundraising leadership of Alice Butler-Short, we were able to raise money for a waterfall and small pond. Initially, we received neither support nor money from the central office of the Whitman-Walker Clinic. They were struggling to keep their clinics open throughout the metropolitan area; they were afraid that our efforts might divert donor dollars from the services they provide. But that didn't stop us. Once we got started, the momentum just kept growing. The healing garden seemed to take on its own energy and life.

I had been afraid that we might not be able to mobilize others to help, but help always appeared when we needed it. Volunteers logged in hundreds of hours—individuals, clubs, and groups. Gays and lesbians worked side by side with heterosexual volunteers, and local businesses and individuals made generous contributions. A group of tree service companies donated their services for a day, trimming branches and removing dead trees and stumps. A neighborhood resident donated a twenty-year-old weeping Japanese maple tree with a one-ton root ball that he had dug up from his yard. After nursing it with water and love for four months, we planted it beside the waterfall. Additional plants would occasionally appear, as people dropped by and put them in the ground.

I give thanks to whatever spirits whispered in my ear today and gently led me through the gate of this very special garden. I will try to carry its energy in my heart and consciousness when I am outside the walls.

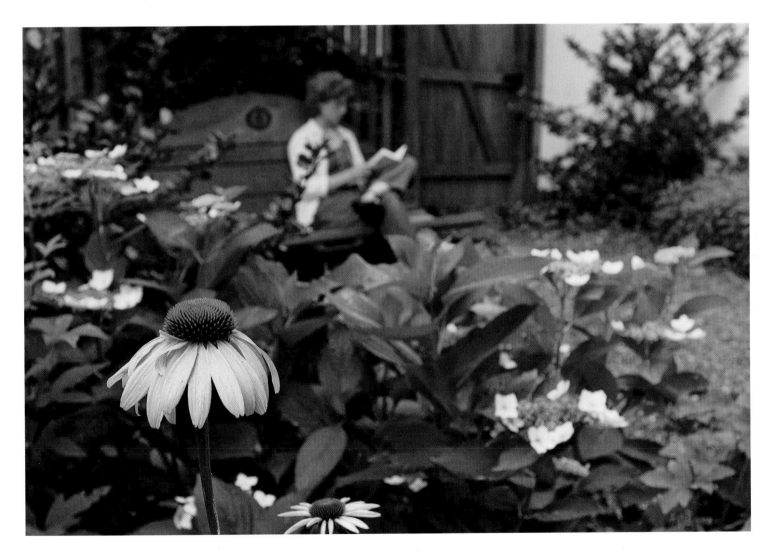

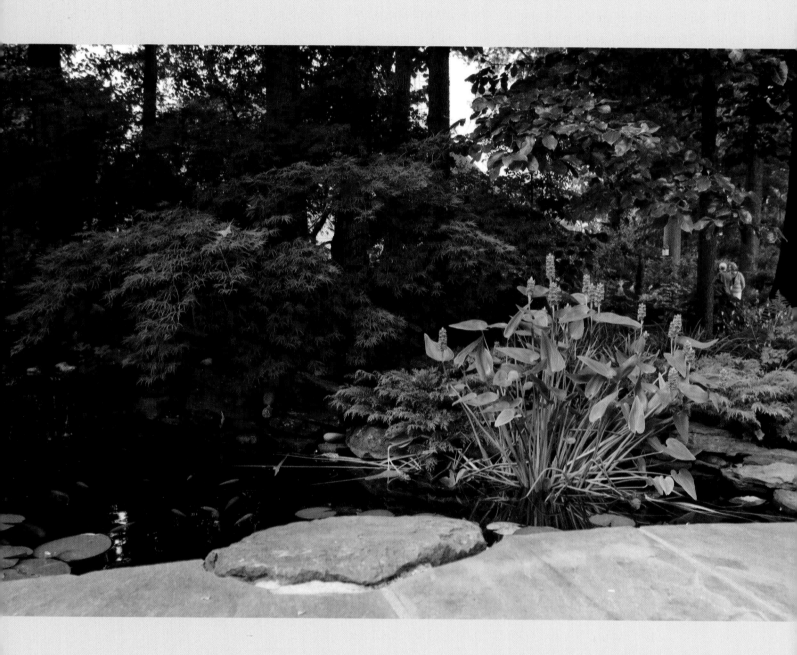

I've always felt that the space has its own magic. We would marvel because the garden is on a very busy, noisy street, but inside, the noise quickly disappears. In terms of garden design, the space feels right. In my business, I've sometimes had to force something on a space because a client wants this or that. But the best gardens are the ones that fit the space. It's important to have a controlling hand, but it's also important to listen to what the garden says it should be—and this garden spoke to us very clearly. I think that all of us who worked on the project feel a sense of wonder at how it came together virtually without conflict, and with every person essential to its success. What exists today, compared with what was in that space when we started, is a miracle. The garden has allowed people—clinic staff, clients, people in the community—to see the power of possibility, and I think that's very important. When people can't see possibilities for change, they get stuck and constrained.

After several years of work, we had converted about two-thirds of the space into a healing garden, completing what we called phase one and phase two. But there was still a large space that was a mess, full of poison ivy and weeds, and there were a lot of things we still needed, including an irrigation system and lights for nighttime use of the garden. Then, right on schedule, something serendipitous happened. A horticulturist who had recently moved to our area went to a conference where he met the folks from TKF, which turned out to be a crucial connection for the completion of the garden. Each time something like this happens, it renews my faith that there's a pattern and a purpose in the universe and that things will work out for the best. We took care of the final details and built the labyrinth, which has been key to bringing people into this space.

Our labyrinth is beautiful and a little different from most others: it has three boulders in the center. To me, they have an anchoring effect and act as a fulcrum of strength. But they also provide a resting place, which is important because some of the people who come to use the labyrinth are ill or weak and need to sit. The boulders were intentionally placed in a symbolic triangle, representing both the gay triangle—a symbol created in Nazi Germany to mark undesirables (the color pink for homosexuals)—and, in a spiritual sense, the Holy Trinity. The three boulders in the center are echoed by three boulders on the outside of the labyrinth, giving a walker the feeling of being held and protected. In fact, I think this feeling of being encompassed and safe is present throughout the whole garden and is probably one of the reasons so many people visit.

One of the requirements for TKF funding was to increase our community outreach. Through our sizeable volunteer base, we had already done a good

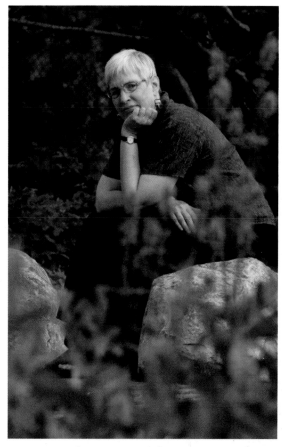

Karen Rowe, Firesoul

Today I begin a new chapter in my life—
a chapter of healing, not from pains,
sickness or wounds,
but from my internal world.
The garden represents peace and comfort.
I come here not to be healed, but to find
purpose in life, and the garden helped.

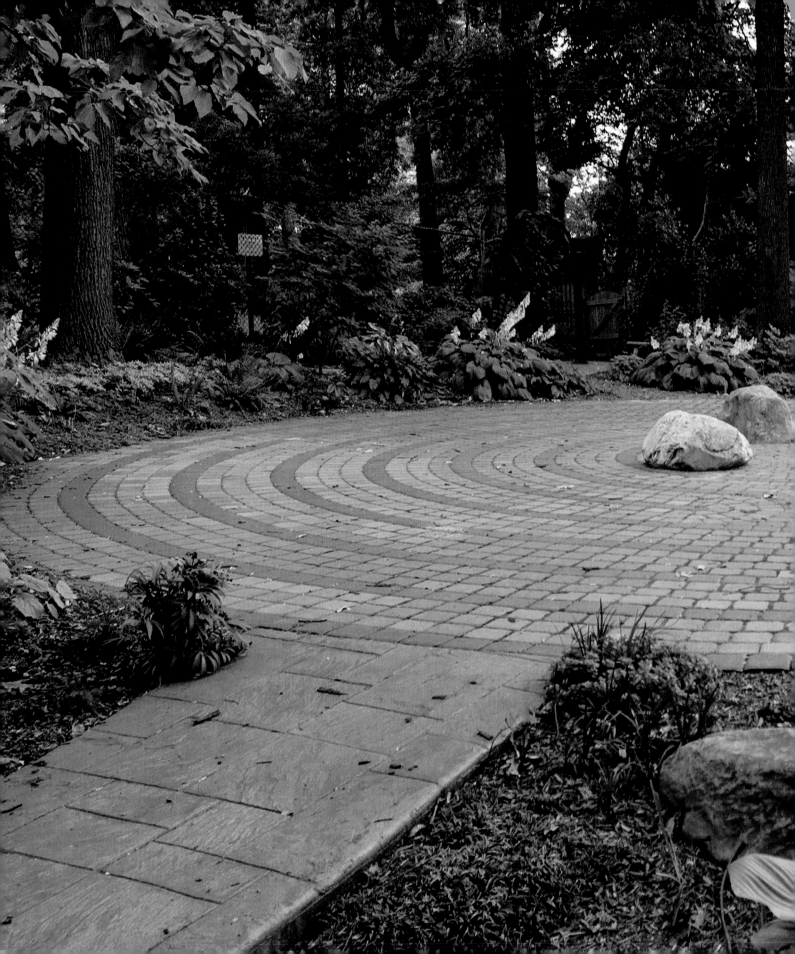

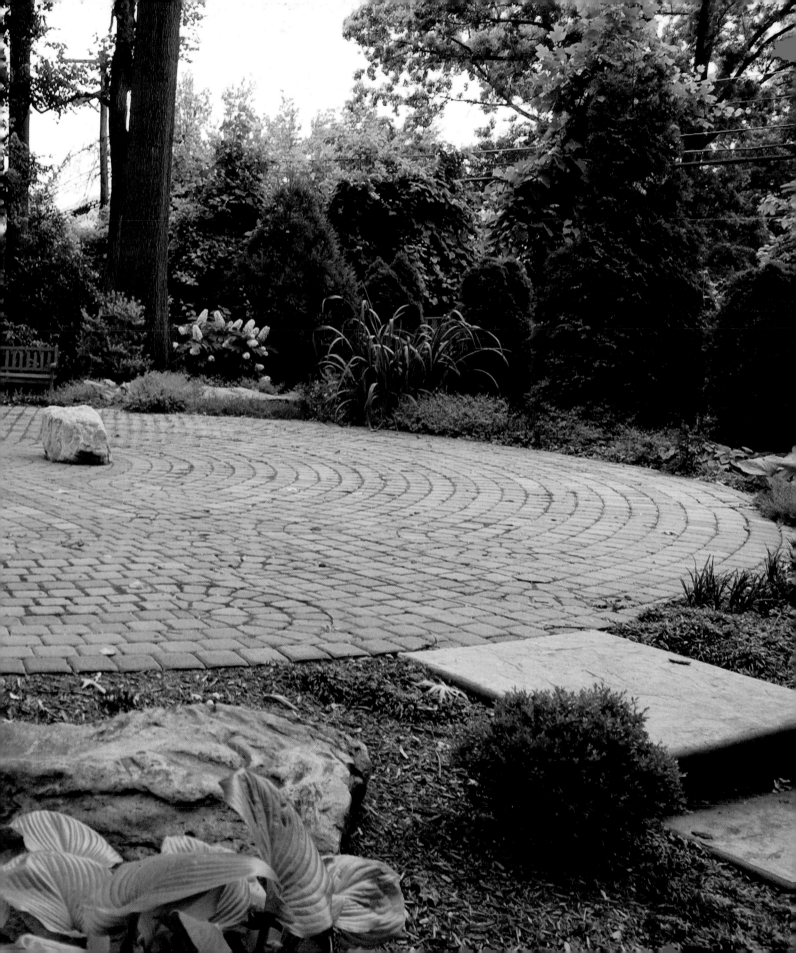

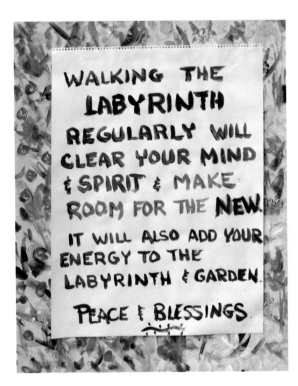

WALKING THE LABYRINTH REGULARLY WILL CLEAR YOUR MIND & SPIRIT & MAKE ROOM FOR THE NEW. IT WILL ALSO ADD YOUR ENERGY TO THE LABYRINTH & GARDEN. PEACE & BLESSINGS.

God, I see your presence everywhere I look. I feel your peace in this beautiful garden. I see your love in my daughter's big brown eyes. I don't feel so lost anymore, but I really need your help dealing with an illness that has no cure.

bit of outreach, but we made a more concerted effort to let people know about the space, by contacting churches and civic organizations. We also partnered with a nearby church that had been offering labyrinth walks for years. We alternated using their labyrinth and ours for organized walks, which introduced new people to our healing garden each time and spread the word. We joined the Labyrinth Society, which has brought people to our garden from all over the surrounding area and from distant places as well. And we found just the right person—Karen Rowe—to be our labyrinth coordinator and help build the bridge that connects the clinic to the community.

Now there is a steady stream of individuals who come to the garden. We keep a simple brochure at the entrance for people who aren't familiar with walking a labyrinth. Karen also welcomes groups and helps them understand how to use the labyrinth as a meditation tool. For example, she was contacted by a local church who wanted to demystify AIDS for its young people. Karen gave them an introduction to the labyrinth, and after they had walked it, the outreach worker from the clinic talked with the teens and gave them good health information that might be hard for them to come by elsewhere. A nearby massage school brings its students, to learn how to use the labyrinth as a resource for themselves, so that they don't burn out once they start practicing. A Latino support group for lesbians meets here every week when it's good weather.

The staff of the clinic also uses the garden. At first, some of the clinic staff members were enamored with the labyrinth, and some weren't. But there came a time when a funding crisis threw the future of the clinic—and the future of their jobs—into uncertainty. Their own anxiety made it harder than usual to deal with the problems and pain of their clients. So Karen, who is also an artist, took a canvas and painted some images of her personal experiences that had come out of the healing garden. She put the canvas on an easel in the reception area and wrote on it, "The labyrinth is your friend. It can help you." That was a turning point for the staff members, who began to appreciate and use the garden and labyrinth more. Today, Karen continues to oversee the space, traveling from her home many miles away to help maintain the garden and organize events. New staff members often tell us that they chose to work at this particular clinic because of the beautiful garden and labyrinth. To think that the garden attracts top-notch, committed employees to the clinic makes me feel really good about the outcome of our efforts.

In addition to the labyrinth, our garden has another unique feature—the sculpture of Caroline Hufford-Anderson. She is a grandmother and a sculptor with an enormous zest for life and people. Soon after her eldest son died

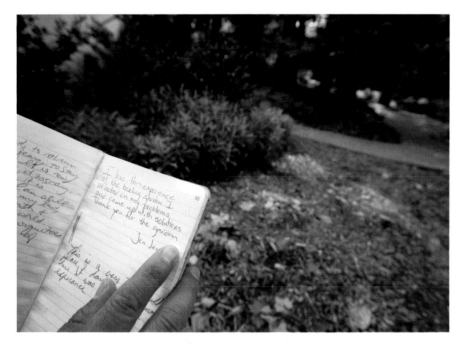

Such a beautiful day. The scents of the garden lifted my heart. On the labyrinth, I gathered up my soul.

of AIDS, she heard about the plans to create a healing garden at the clinic, and she became one of the project's most passionate advocates. As visitors approach the labyrinth, they encounter her sculpture *David's Gate.* The six-feet-high wrought-iron sculpture symbolizes the biblical story of King David, who was devastated with grief at the death of his son Absalom. With its gateway shaped in the form of a human ribcage, the sculpture stands as a metaphor for moving through grief to acceptance. I think the sculpture touches everyone who sees it simply because the theme of loss is universal— as is the desire to be healed and whole.

Certainly my experience in helping to create the garden has been healing for me. It has made me a believer in coming together with other people for the common good. At the time I became involved with the garden, my partner was battling a lung disease that eventually took his life. Working on a project that was close to my heart helped me a lot. I was able to be open with people who had experienced the same kind of losses, and every time I worked as a volunteer, I felt better. I connected with people's goodness in every interaction, and I learned a lesson that I've carried with me ever since: if I start feeling sad, the best antidote is to go out and help others.

I walked in, burdened and confused.
I walked around, letting go.
I stood in the center, illuminated by guidance and understanding.
I walked out, light, loved, and loving.

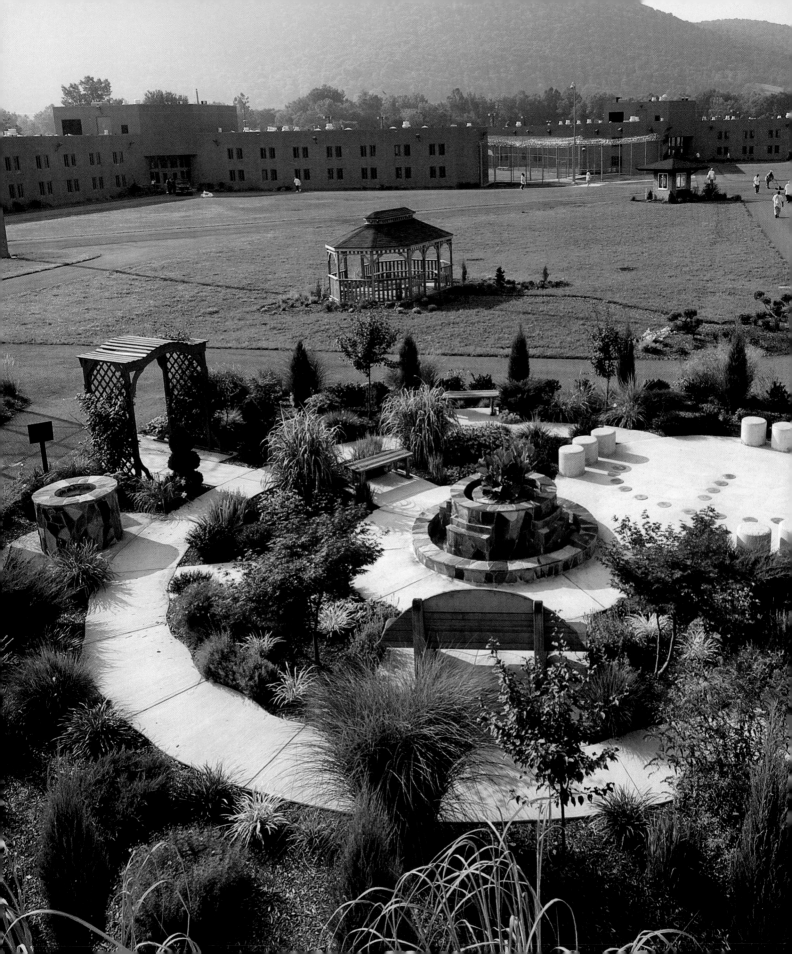

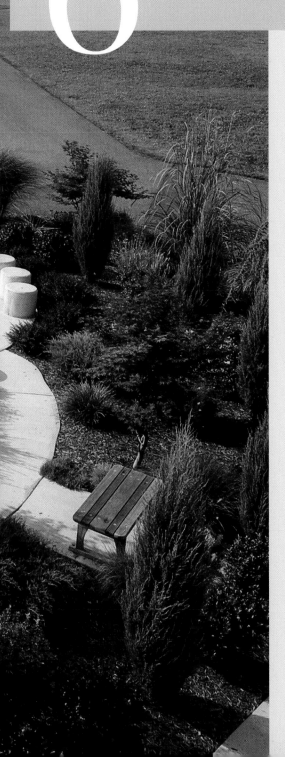

6 Meditation Garden at the Western Correctional Institution

One of the inmates said to me, 'I've done a lot of destructive things in my life. Making this garden is a chance for me to do something positive.' I think that's why they take such good care of the garden. It's a place that honors their humanity in an environment where they have to put on their emotional armor to survive.

—Tony Lawlor, Firesoul

In the United States, there are more than 2.2 million individuals in prison. This country has the highest imprisonment percentage of any nation in the world. In fact, there are more people in U.S. prisons than there are people living in eleven individual states.

One such prison is the Western Correctional Institution (WCI) in Cumberland, Maryland—home to 1,782 inmates and staff members. Here, there are many walls: not just those of barbed wire and stone that surround the area, but also inner walls of fear and loss. Inside a prison, there is no place to be alone to confront those inner walls, no moment to experience just a sliver of human dignity.

At WCI, a very special team of men came together to give this concern their full attention. Jon Galley, WCI's warden, recognized that many of the prisoners under his supervision would one day return home. He wanted to offer them an opportunity to heal and to learn before they got out. Jon enlisted the help of Tony Lawlor, an architect who came to believe that the design for this special space needed to come from the users, the prisoners themselves.

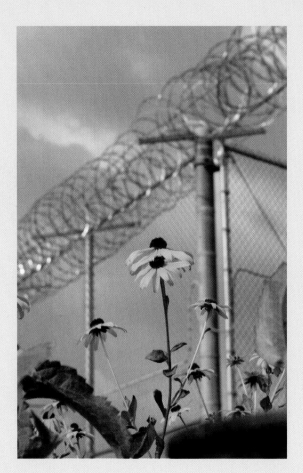

Bill Jewell signed on as the project coordinator and developed techniques to realize a complex project within the tricky confines of a prison setting. Wayne Yoder, a professor of biology living nearby, spent countless hours tilling and planting with the prisoners.

Together they created a meditation garden at WCI. Today, it is the one location where the inmates are free to let down their guard and take in nature, the one spot where they can feel safe long enough to consider letting go of the past, so that they can feel a sense of self-worth and dignity.

Building a garden like this in a prison setting offered a unique set of challenges. First, state law dictates that government dollars cannot be used to fund construction or maintenance of such a space, so money needed to be raised. In addition, eighteen religions are practiced at WCI, and many inmates practice no religion at all; so the design had to be free of all dogma. The architect solved this problem by focusing on nature, including the universal essential element of water.

The U.S. Department of Justice reports that over two-thirds of released prisoners are rearrested within three years. The hope at WCI is that by focusing on the well-being of the prisoners, by introducing them to a new set of skills, both physical and mental, these inmates will never find themselves blocked by these walls again.

—*T.S.*

Jon Galley

Former Warden, Western Correctional Institution

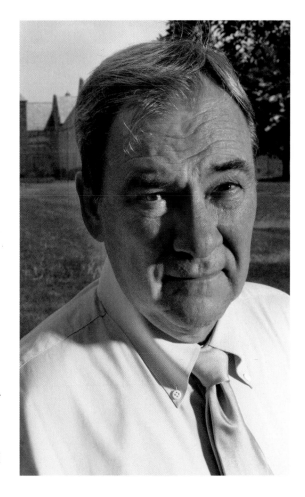

I've always been a believer in the impact of environment on people. I think the best correctional system is one that strikes a balance between the discipline we need to have and a softer environment that encourages something different, a more human side. Of course, not everyone agrees with me. Some people think that inmates should pay for what they did in every way possible, but I just don't see any reason why a prison has to look stark and cold, like a 1920s stone bastion. I don't think there's anything wrong with pictures on the walls, carpets on the floors, and flowers on the grounds. In fact, you can track my career in corrections from institution to institution by the flower beds, ornamental trees, and shrubs on the prison grounds.

One of the first things I wanted to do when I became warden of the Western Correctional Institution in 1999 was make it beautiful, and I wanted to put the inmates to work doing that. But what happened at WCI when we connected with the TKF Foundation blossomed into something far beyond what I had expected—and a lot quicker than I could have imagined.

I was lucky on two counts. The first was to have Bill Jewell working for me. He wears a lot of hats and is one of the finest employees I've ever had. All I had to do was tell Bill what I wanted and then get out of the way. The stars must have been aligned. When I talked to Bill about beautifying the compound, he told me that a biology professor from a nearby university, Wayne Yoder, had just applied to become a volunteer. That's how we got our Master Gardener program started, and the amount of time Wayne has put into it year after year is astonishing.

Within a couple of years, the compound looked completely different. We gave the inmates in the horticulture program pretty much free rein to create whatever they wanted. We didn't tell them to lay out a bed this way or that way. The only thing I said was that I didn't want straight lines or box-shaped

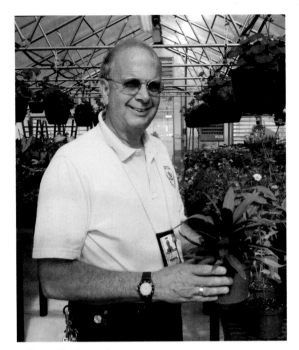
Bill Jewell, Firesoul

beds. "Use your imagination," I told them, and they did. The gardens have swirls and circles and all kinds of shapes.

The program was so successful that we decided we needed a greenhouse where we could grow our own plants. We knew we wouldn't get state money for it, so we started to explore the possibility of getting funding from a foundation. Wayne connected with TKF, but found out that they don't fund greenhouses. However, they were intrigued with our gardening program. They told us if we were interested in creating a meditation garden, they would fund it and a greenhouse as well.

Once we started to think about a meditation garden, the need for such a place became quite evident. While inmates are cut off from the rest of the world, and alone in that sense, they are never alone in the prison. They are housed two to a cell, and most of their time is spent in a variety of group activities. Before the garden, there was no place for solitude; there was no place they could be by themselves in a time of family crisis. Inmates can't leave to attend a funeral if a mother or father or other loved one passes away. They

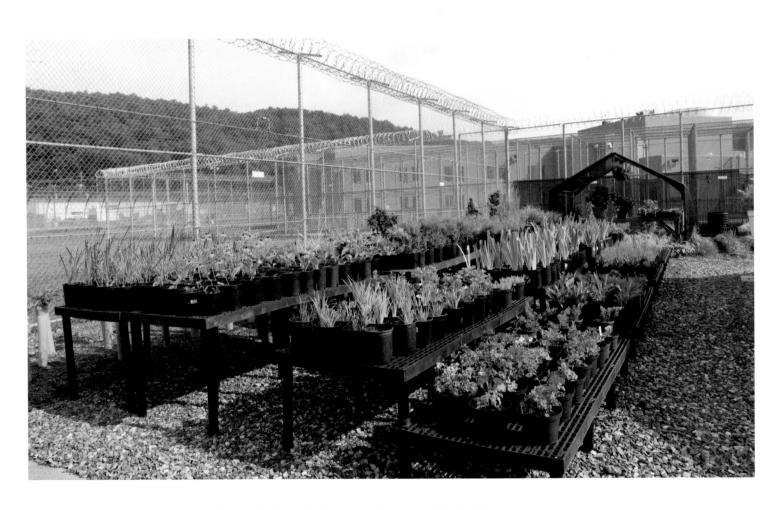

can't celebrate joyous occasions, like graduations and weddings, with their families. So we saw the garden as a place for inmates to be alone to grieve. We saw it as a place for them to reflect on their lives and what they would like them to be, inside the prison or outside it, after they are released.

All three of us—Wayne, Bill, and myself—were committed to making the meditation garden happen, and TKF brought in an architect to help with the design. But it took nothing short of a miracle to pull off a construction project of this magnitude in a prison that was in full use the whole time. Bill Jewell was the miracle worker.

Security was a top priority for us, so that none of the tools or equipment could be used to escape or to harm other people. The first thing Bill did was construct a twelve-foot-high security fence around the site of the garden and assign staff to guard the area. He put razor wire at the top of the fence, and the gate into the site was kept locked at all times. We brought backhoes into the area. A big truck, which usually drills holes for telephone poles, came in to drill holes for the circular concrete benches. Cement trucks came in and out to pour concrete. A well-driller drilled the hole for the twenty-foot-long steel pipe that's in the Well of Unspoken Truths. Then trucks full of stones were brought in, and a masonry contractor built the well. One of the female staff members in the fiscal office helped with the stonework. All the vehicles came in through a special gate, each one was searched, and guards inspected the undersides with mirrors. And that's how WCI came to be the only correctional institution in the country, that I'm aware of anyway, with a meditation garden.

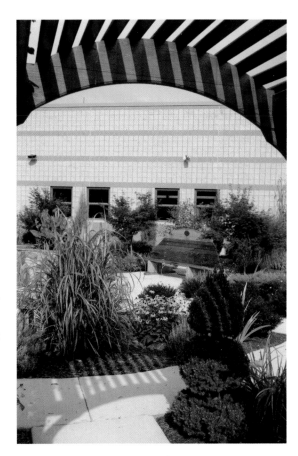

I'm a gardener myself. I love flowers, but even more I like the environment they create: a place where people can lose themselves. The inmates, as crass and hard as they want to appear to be, may not admit that it does something for them to sit in the meditation garden with flowers around them. But you can see that it does make a difference. They're careful in the garden. They don't abuse it. They stay on the walkways. There aren't paths cut through the beds or the grass at WCI, and the inmates don't tear up the shrubs and flowers as I've seen them do at other institutions. That's partly because we wouldn't tolerate it, but it's also because they take pride in the garden—especially the men who worked on it. A lot of the inmates come from places that were noth-ing but concrete and blacktop. Many of them didn't know how to push a lawn-mower or how to use a rake or shovel. Now they look at what they've created, and they are very proud of their work—as well they should be. It's gorgeous.

We have about 1,700 inmates, and some of them are never going to be released. That's one reason I think the environment and meditation garden are important. This is all they'll see for the rest of their lives. The other reason is that about 90 percent of the inmates *will* be released back into society. I think it behooves us to soften their environment, because I believe it softens them.

I joke with the inmates in the greenhouse that the first marijuana plant I find in there is going to be a big problem for them. Sooner or later, it's going to happen. But that's not a good reason not to have a greenhouse or gardens. These guys have twenty-four hours a day to think, which is why we've always had and always will have security concerns. But a system has to balance its discipline with something gentler, because we're dealing with human beings.

I've often thought that the thing an employee in our business has to be most concerned with is getting jaded about human nature. God knows we deal with some really bad people that have done and continue to do very bad things. I don't pretend that we cure any of them. I lost that notion a long time ago. I do, however, think we should try to expose them to whatever it is that will make something click and keep them out of prison. It's hard to track inmates once they leave, but I know of one who has started his own landscaping business. For a lot of the prisoners, being involved in the horticulture program and the garden was the first time in their life they did anything that worked. It might just be the thing that keeps them from coming back.

Greetings. Do not let the world distract you. Focus within. New beginnings. Start within.

Today I became someone different. I made something very special come alive. A place built where we could sit, think, and get outside and get our minds together. To be a part of something like this is wonderful, and I am glad to be a part of this garden.

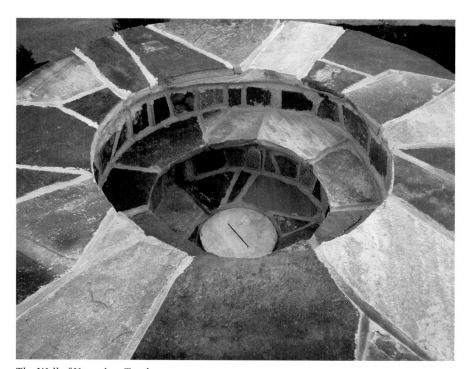

The Well of Unspoken Truths

Tony Lawlor

Architect

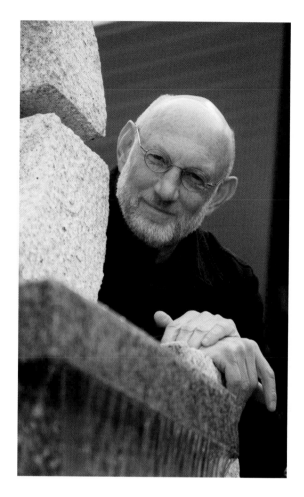

The TKF Foundation contacted me about seven years ago because of a book I had written called *The Temple in the House: Finding the Sacred in Everyday Architecture*. It deals with the idea that the structures we create around us are reflections of our inner psychological and emotional experiences. TKF began using the book as a guide for people who were doing projects with them, and they invited me to help design the meditation garden at the Western Correctional Institution. I jumped at the chance to be involved in such a unique project—but I never could have imagined how deeply it would affect me and influence my work.

As I approached the WCI, which is situated in the beautiful Cumberland Valley of Maryland, I became immediately aware of the natural beauty surrounding the facility and began to think of how we might connect the garden within the prison to the natural garden all around it.

It had already been decided that one of the purposes of the garden would be to provide a place of solitude for inmates to grieve the loss of a loved one and to reflect. So the first step for me was to use a process of visioning that I use with all my clients. We brought together a group that included some of the inmates in the horticulture program, Wayne Yoder, Bill Jewell, the chaplain, the warden, a TKF staff member, some security officers, and myself. I began by asking the inmates if they had ever been to a place they considered a meditation garden, and each one of them said yes. They hadn't called it a meditation garden, but it was a place they used to decompress: a park, a fountain by the Chesapeake Bay, a bench under a tree. I wanted the meditation garden to be a reflection of what was important and meaningful to them, so I had them close their eyes, and I asked them questions that I hoped would call forth images.

The first image that came up was a circle, and that became the shape of the garden. Another image was water. The sound of water was important too.

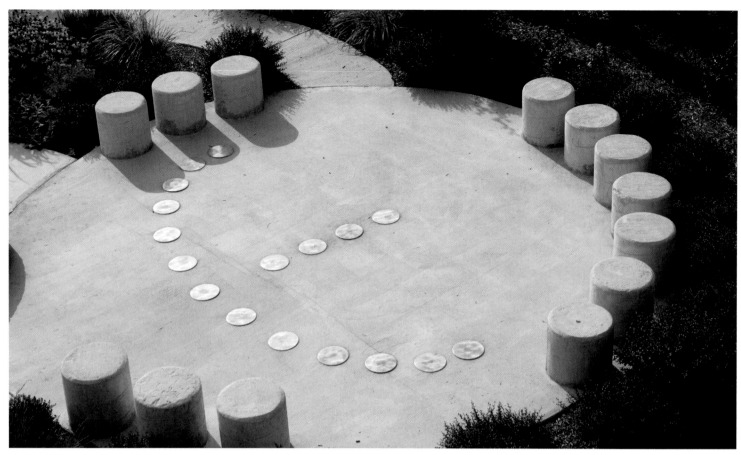

Human sundial

A place for thought
A place for bliss
A place to reflect on the past
A place to contemplate the future

We got more specific with the idea of a tree in the center of a well with water flowing out in all four directions. That image became the center focus of the garden. I talked to them about different concepts in architecture. The gate, for example, often traditionally meets at twin pillars, and passing through a gate can represent both hope and fear. We explored that further, and I asked them what they hoped for. They said, "To get out of prison." Then I asked them what they feared, and they said, "Getting out of prison." The gate in their garden is an arbor that you walk through. They took it one step further and planted red roses climbing up one side to symbolize the constant struggle with violence and white roses climbing up the other to symbolize the hope for peace. The roses have now grown to the point where the red and the white meet at the top of the arbor: it makes a striking impression.

Another feature of the garden that came out of this visioning session was the Well of Unspoken Truths. In addition to the central well, we have a smaller circular masonry well off to one side. We sank a steel pipe twenty feet long into the ground in the center of the well, sealed it, and put a small slit at the top, so that inmates can write on pieces of paper and drop them into the well without fear that anyone else will read them. In this way, the inmates can express thoughts and feelings that are inside of them but would make them too vulnerable if revealed. We have benches, some wood and some concrete, so that groups have a place to gather or inmates can talk to the chaplain. There is also a large sundial, embedded in the ground, big enough for a person to stand in and cast the shadow that tells time. It seemed symbolic—they're doing time, so why not be time? In addition, the image of time in a circular pattern has a wholeness to it, enabling an inmate to connect to a time before he was in prison and to a time when he will be out.

The process of designing the garden took on a life of its own, and one of my greatest lessons learned was to listen deeply to what the inmates wanted. There were times in the beginning when I thought, "Wow, this is a great opportunity to do something really clever or something visually interesting." But every time I tried it on paper, it just seemed fake. Many of the people who hire an architect have a lot of money and are concerned about self-image, about perpetuating a front that they want to present to the world. But here I was working with guys who had nothing to lose. Their level of directness and honesty in working together really opened my mind and heart, an unexpected gift that I have carried with me ever since, in my work and in my life.

One of the most amazing experiences, for me, happened at one of the planning meetings. The whole cast of characters was there, from security officers to inmates. We were talking about plants. There was a moment when all the roles fell away, and we were just a bunch of people talking about what plants would be best for the garden. Working on this project blasted open my preconceived ideas of what inmates are like. Several of them thanked me for listening to them and for letting them make the garden what they wanted. In doing so, we gave them the opportunity to see the power of their own creativity. One of the inmates said to me, "I've done a lot of destructive things in my life. This is a way I can do something positive." I think that's why they take such good care of the garden. It's a place that honors their humanity in an environment where they have to put on their emotional armor to survive.

Another gift for me was being part of a team that was absolutely, unequivocally committed to making this garden happen. Warden Galley said, "We're going to get this garden built no matter what." Wayne Yoder's commitment to the inmates and his steady presence in the prison were remarkable. And Bill Jewell performed miracle after miracle of logistics, getting everything from trucks to concrete to dangerous tools into the prison.

Whenever I tell people about this garden, they are incredibly inspired. I think that's because at some level they understand right away that what we

Thank you, Lord, for the sacred space Thou hast provided, making a paradise of these prison walls.

In the midst of pain, anger, and frustration, this is an oasis of calm and beauty. God, thank you for small things.

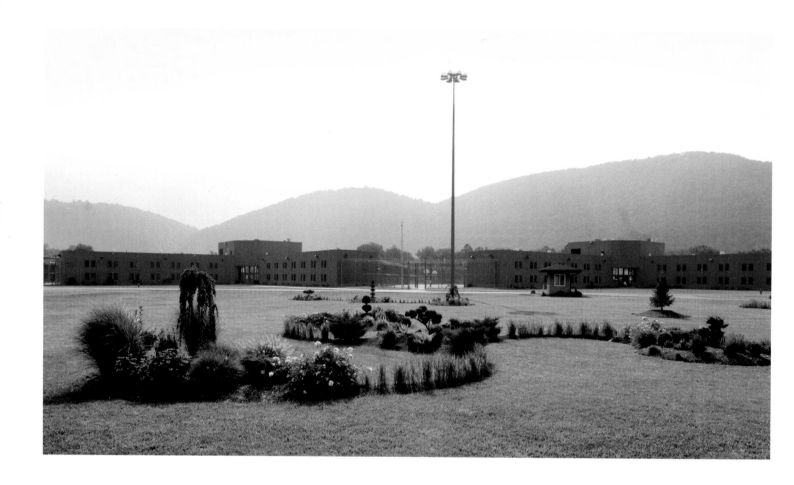

Through the mountainside's gentle pull, the breeze stirring the garden's stillness opens a doorway within. Thank you, Lord, for the privilege of life.

created in the prison is a metaphor for life. We all live within boundaries that can sometimes be oppressive—taxes, bills, work, relationships, illness—and within these limitations, we seek to find places of sanctuary, whether it's a place in the physical world or a quiet center within ourselves. A garden in a prison is a concrete example of that—a garden that blooms within a space that is fenced and topped with razor wire. The inmates chose to put a circle in the midst of an environment that is mostly rectangular and boxy. They created a little opening in the grid of their lives to find their moment of peace and freedom. Isn't that what we all want to do?

Wayne Yoder

Professor of Biology and WCI Volunteer

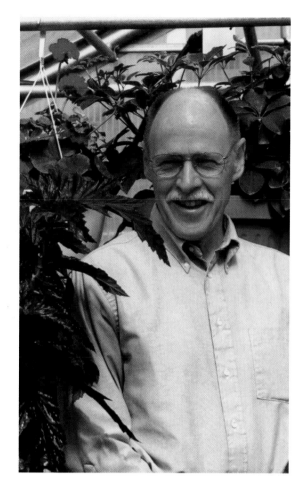

My parents taught me not to complain about a situation unless I was willing to do something to make it better. That was my motivation for becoming a volunteer at the Western Correctional Institution in 1999. I was bothered by the fact that prison populations kept getting larger and larger, that the State of Maryland kept building more prisons to accommodate them, and that there didn't seem to be any end in sight. WCI was about ten minutes from my house, so I went over and volunteered to do whatever they thought may help to reduce recidivism.

It seems that I walked in at just the right moment. Warden Galley had just given Bill Jewell the responsibility of beautifying the grounds. When Bill heard that I was a biology professor, he asked me if I'd teach a horticulture class. I hesitated slightly—biology and horticulture are not the same thing. But I'm a gardener who grew up on a farm, and I know and teach about insect pests and fungus diseases, so I said yes. I thought that maybe I could help the inmates learn some gardening and landscaping skills that would be useful when they got out of prison and that could help them stay out. But what we've learned from one another by working together over the years goes far beyond gardening skills.

One of the first things I did was design a couple of plantings. The beds had already been dug, so I designed the gardens and chose the plants. Then I worked side by side with the inmates to plant the beds. Those were the first and last beds I designed; the inmates planned and designed the rest. We bought the plants for the first five beds in the compound from local nurseries—and it's important to clarify that we didn't buy anything using tax dollars. We used the "inmate welfare fund," which is the profit that comes from the sale of goods in the commissary.

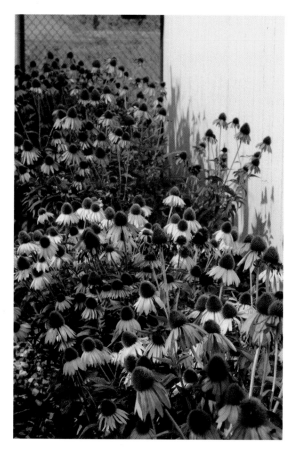

Designing the plantings for the compound required a level of complexity unlike anything else I have ever experienced. Because of the security restrictions, we can't grow anything greater than a certain height and a certain width, and anytime a security officer has a concern about something getting in the way, we prune. Last year we had to cut back a plant that a guard said was obstructing a camera a hundred yards away! Tools are another issue. There are plenty of garden tools that could be used as weapons if someone chose to—picks, hammers, shovels, rakes. But we have them all because Warden Galley and Bill Jewell agreed that the garden is worth the risk. Everything is inventoried and kept on a tool board in the shed. Horticulture inmates have access to tools during the day; every night, tools are inventoried, and the shed is locked.

As we prepared to continue the beautification project with landscaping around the four inmate housing units and the guard shacks, we realized how useful it would be to have our own greenhouse, not only to grow our own stock but also to provide horticulture jobs for some inmates. I located three used greenhouses for sale, but for one reason or another, none of them panned out—which turned out to be a stroke of good fortune. It forced us to go looking for foundation money to build a greenhouse, and after searching dozens of Web sites, I discovered the TKF Foundation. Except that we couldn't have our greenhouse unless we built a meditation garden! That seemed fine to me, because I believe strongly in the value of meditation. But the truth is, we really didn't have a clue what TKF had been doing or what would happen at WCI

Respect each man's walk in life—no matter that you may not have any understanding of it.

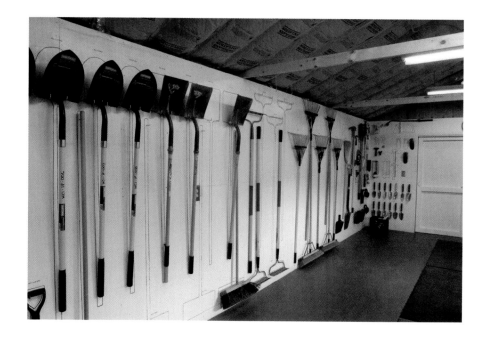

when they brought in an architect to work with us. The project we embarked on went far beyond what Bill Jewell and I had imagined.

I believe that one person can make a difference, and my time working with the inmates has strengthened that belief. But the meditation garden also demonstrated what amazing feats can be accomplished by teamwork. All of us at WCI and TKF worked together to make the garden happen. My role on the team was—and continues to be—to help the inmates grow the plants for the garden. It gives me a way to work with them, to teach them horticulture and gardening, and to perhaps open them to a wider view of possibilities. Certainly, one of the gifts for me was to gain a much better understanding of who the inmates are.

In all the time I've been here, I've never had a bad experience. I try to live my life by the golden rule, so at the prison, I always start off by saying, "I'm here to work with you as a person. I'll treat you no differently than if we were on the outside." I don't ask the inmates why they are in prison or how long their sentence is. Some of them have told me, but I never ask. I treat them with respect, and they have always treated me the same way. One thing I've come to appreciate is that despite the bad choices they have made in their lives, they are still human beings. Now they're paying a penalty for those choices, but they are still human. I try to encourage them to think about their situation and to help them see that they can still do good things, even though they are in prison.

One way to show them respect is to give them as much freedom as possible in their very confining environment. For example, there are a number of different kinds of theme gardens that I would like to have seen in the compound—native Maryland plants, for one—but I've let go of that. The responsibility for designing the compound and the plantings in the meditation garden is entirely theirs, and seeing the pride they take in their work is a much greater reward than seeing a garden of my own favorite plants. It's amazing what they come up with. They have access to catalogs, so they can see the kinds of things we might be able to grow. One of the men has a very good eye for plantings. He puts things together on paper, and then we grow the plants in the greenhouse and plant his designs.

Another form of freedom for inmates is being outside. Prisoners in the horticulture program get to spend a lot of time outdoors. It can get extremely hot in this valley in the summer. There was one day when the temperature was predicted to go up to ninety-five degrees. I had a meeting somewhere else that afternoon, but I made it clear to the men that I didn't expect them to continue to work in the heat. One of them looked at me and said, "I'd rather be out

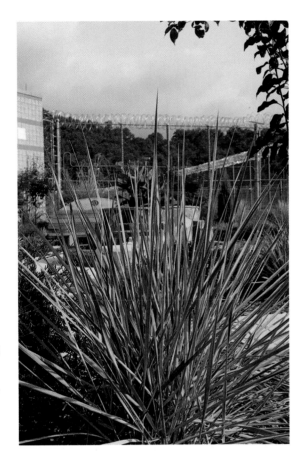

This is a peaceful place, a place where I can lay my hair down; but there's a serious problem—I don't have any hair (smile).

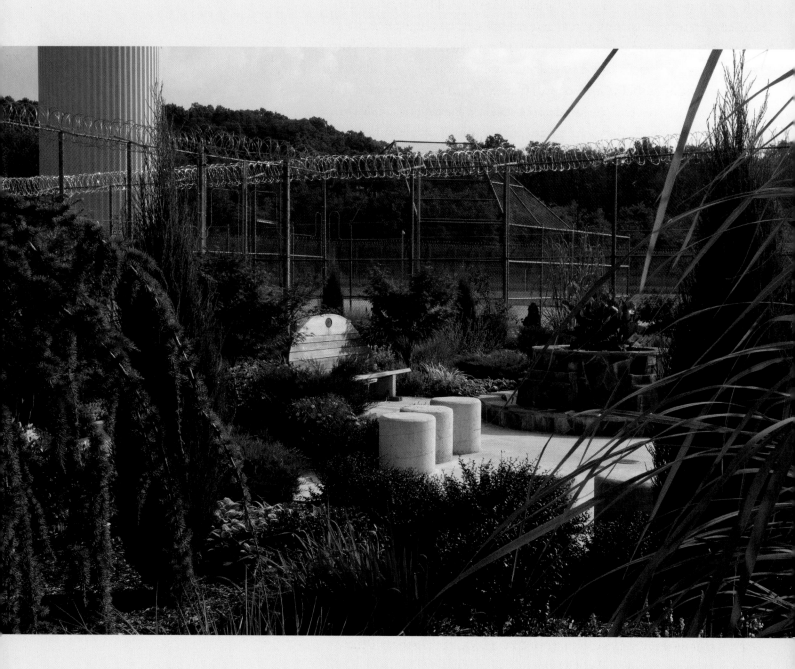

here working in the heat than in my cell." Every one of them worked through the afternoon. Knowing how important it was for them to be outside made a real impression on me—especially when a lifer gave his space in the horticulture program to another inmate. He said, "I'd love to be the one out in the yard, but he's going to get out of here, and he can use the experience he'll get." I thought that was tremendous. This individual was looking out for somebody else even though he really wanted that experience for himself.

One thing I was told when I started volunteering in the prison was not to become friends with any of the inmates, because it is against prison rules to do favors for anyone. Everyone has to be treated equally. That's hard, because I've come to appreciate some of the men almost as friends. When we were planning the beds around the housing units, one of the inmates asked me if it was wrong for him to request certain plants in front of his window. I thought about it and decided that would not be considered a special favor. So he took the initiative and planted some fragrant things that he can smell in the summer when his window is open. He didn't explain his choices to me, but I've wondered if the scents he chose connect him to a garden or a person in his life outside prison.

The inmates have taught me what it's like to be free, as opposed to being confined, and I'm so grateful for that. It won't be too long until I retire, and I could very well enjoy spending more time here. One of the most well-known scriptures from the Bible asks, "What does the Lord require of you? To seek justice and love mercy and to walk humbly with your God." What I do at the prison is show a little mercy to men that need something to brighten their lives. I can do that while I'm teaching horticulture and not make a big deal of it.

Every once in a while, I get to see a life transformed. One of the inmates told me that he came from a city and that the experience of gardening—of working in the soil and planting seeds and learning about plant diseases—had totally opened him up. Because of what he had learned in class, he was seeing for the first time in his life the beauty of the natural world, including the lovely mountains that surround the prison. He said, "I have a whole new appreciation, and when I get out of here, the world's going to be so different than it was when I came in." Most of these men are going to be somebody's neighbor sometime in the future. The more we can do to help them be good, productive neighbors, the better it'll be for all of us.

To those who I've hurt: I'm sorry.
To those who I've lost: You are missed.

A quiet place! My soul grows still. This indeed is a balm for the weary, a shelter for the beaten. I am so grateful for this quiet place. I am now renewed.

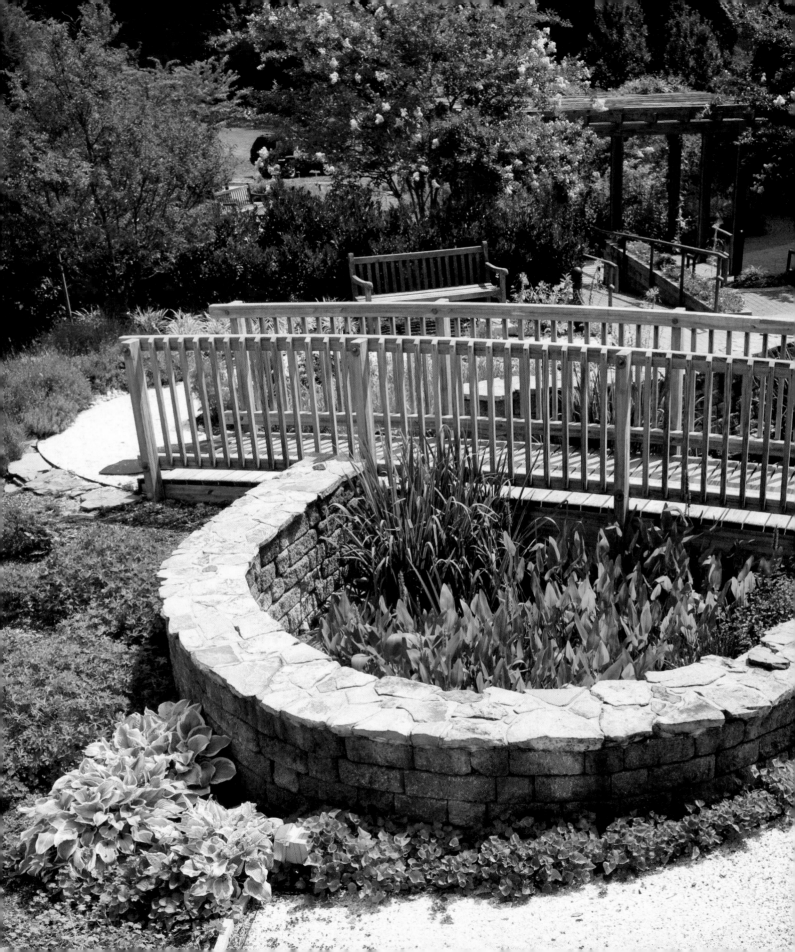

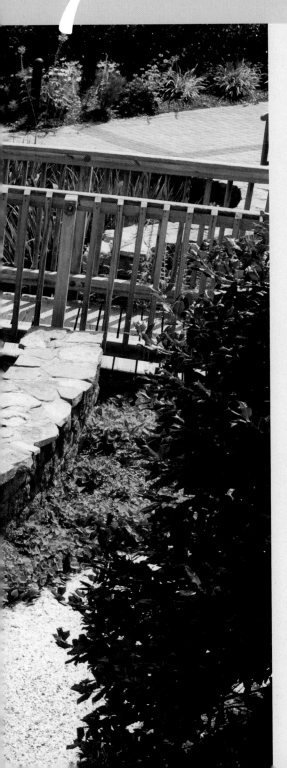

7 Therapeutic Healing Garden at Kernan Hospital

A study has been done that compared two groups of hospital patients, and the people who looked at trees used less pain medication, felt less stress, and had lower blood pressure.

—Linda Hutchinson-Troyer, Firesoul

The Neuro-Rehabilitation Units at Kernan Hospital in Baltimore remind us that life can change in an instant. Patients arrive at Kernan after a devastating accident or illness has irrevocably altered their lives. Some have suffered a stroke. Others are transferred directly from the area's shock trauma unit, where they have undergone surgical procedures for life-threatening injuries. At Kernan, they must relearn the basic functions of talking and walking. Some must learn how to live confined to a wheelchair.

Linda Hutchinson-Troyer is the patient therapy manager for the Neuro-Rehabilitation Units. As a recreational therapist, she has spent her career working in an environment that looks at the interrelationship between the mind and the body. Her training has been to rehabilitate individuals through specialized activities, and her experience has shown her that the physical environment greatly affects a patient's ability to heal. Today there is mounting research in the health-care field to back up her personal observations. Evidence-based design—architecture based on the emotional and physical needs of the patient—has been found to have a significant influence on recovery. This confirmed Linda's own experience as a gardener who grew up surrounded by flowers, vegetables, and fruit trees at her family home in Pennsylvania. "Gardens help keep people healthy," she believes.

The Kernan administration supported Linda's efforts to raise funds for a garden on the hospital grounds. The leaders listened to her impassioned call, and they in turn became a catalyst for others, by involving the greater community in creating the healing qualities of this space. The local garden club, the Boy Scouts, community youth, and former patients—all played major roles in the process of building the many layers of hope this garden now brings to patients, families, and staff members.

Beyond the basic challenges of realizing the resources to create the space, building a garden in this setting also required special design considerations. Hidden in the beauty of this garden are rehabilitation tools designed to bring people back to their lives and the things that they love. Every aspect of the garden—from the height of the flowerbeds to the color of the plantings to the angle of the paths—was planned to support patients' recovery. Here, patients find not only a respite in the beauty of nature, but also the tools they need to reenter the world.

—T.S.

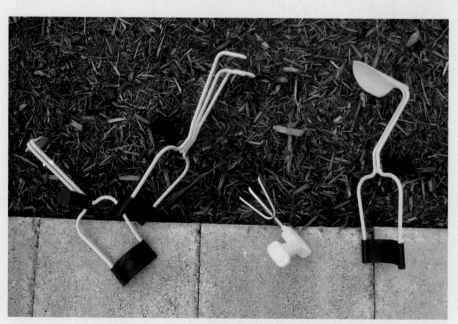

Adaptive gardening tools

Linda Hutchinson-Troyer

Patient Therapy Manager, Kernan Rehabilitation Hospital

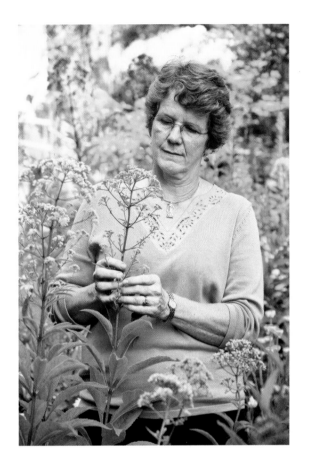

Our healing garden project started as a result of me going to a conference on therapeutic recreation some years ago. I visited the healing garden at the conference site and was very disappointed. It was mostly cement, stainless steel, and brick walls around some holly bushes; it seemed more like a cityscape. My first thought was, "I could do better than this." Then I began to think about the space at the back of Kernan Hospital and how it could be transformed into something really wonderful for our patients.

I enjoy gardening, and, as a recreational therapist, I understand its value. My own roots in gardening go all the way back to the huge garden my parents had at our home in Pennsylvania, where they grew vegetables and flowers, including my father's beautiful rose garden. We even had fruit trees. As an adult, I find working in my own yard very therapeutic. There is plenty of literature that supports the significance of outdoor spaces and how they can help soothe the mind and body.

We all do activities that make us feel good about ourselves—gardening, sports, card games, embroidery, and so on. But imagine your life changing in an instant because of an injury or stroke. Imagine if you felt you couldn't do the things you loved anymore. Your mood and your attitude would plummet; you'd get depressed. Recreational therapists use leisure activities to help rehabilitate patients. We help people see that they can still do the things they love—differently and within their new limitations, but they can still do them. We ask patients, "What did you enjoy doing before your injury or stroke that gave you a sense of satisfaction and well-being?"

At Kernan, we have patients who have suffered brain injury, spinal cord injury, and stroke, as well as people with orthopedic issues like hip and knee

My wish is that any who find this verse may taste this same peace and know creation is all around us, though we ourselves may be in the midst of turmoil, pain, or loss.

replacements. We frequently deal with pain management, and we know that if we can get patients involved in something they like doing, they often forget about their pain and discomfort, at least for a little while. A healing garden would provide patients, especially those who were gardeners, with a beautiful, familiar environment to lift their mood. And for patients who stay at the hospital long enough, we could use a garden as part of their rehabilitation, teaching them how to garden again, through the use of special beds and adaptive tools.

I always like to find a project above and beyond my daily responsibilities to throw myself into. Creating the Kernan healing garden became my project —and my passion—for the next two years. I came back from the conference and went immediately to talk to the hospital's CEO. Just by coincidence, the Ten Hills Garden Club, which has been involved with the hospital for years, had approached him about doing a project only days before. "Why don't you work with the garden club?" he suggested. And I did. The garden club had gotten a grant from the TKF Foundation to create a butterfly garden, and we started with that. We had a limited amount of money, and that turned out to be a good thing—because it motivated us to reach out into the community and pull a lot of people into the project.

The women in the Ten Hills Garden Club were a blessing. One is a biology teacher, and another is chair of the sociology and anthropology program at a nearby university. We put our heads together and got a grant for a program that would involve kids who were at risk; we would use the garden to teach them science and math skills. "Camp Kernan" lasted two weeks. The kids came to the hospital and learned job readiness skills, such as being on time and dressing appropriately. They also learned about rehabilitation. We had some spinal cord injury patients talk to the kids about what it's like to need someone to help you get dressed every day and take you to the bathroom. It was a sort of "scared straight" approach: we wanted to make sure the kids would think twice about drinking and driving.

At the same time, the biology teacher oversaw the creation of the butterfly garden. She taught the kids how to test the soil for alkalinity and acidity. They learned related job skills, including how to use a tiller, how to lay things out, and how to neutralize soil. They learned what mulch is, how to excavate for a path and put down an erosion blanket, and how to tamp down stone dust. Then someone from our integrative medicine program walked the grounds with the kids and showed them different plants that have healing powers. In those two weeks, the butterfly garden was created. It was a win-win situation.

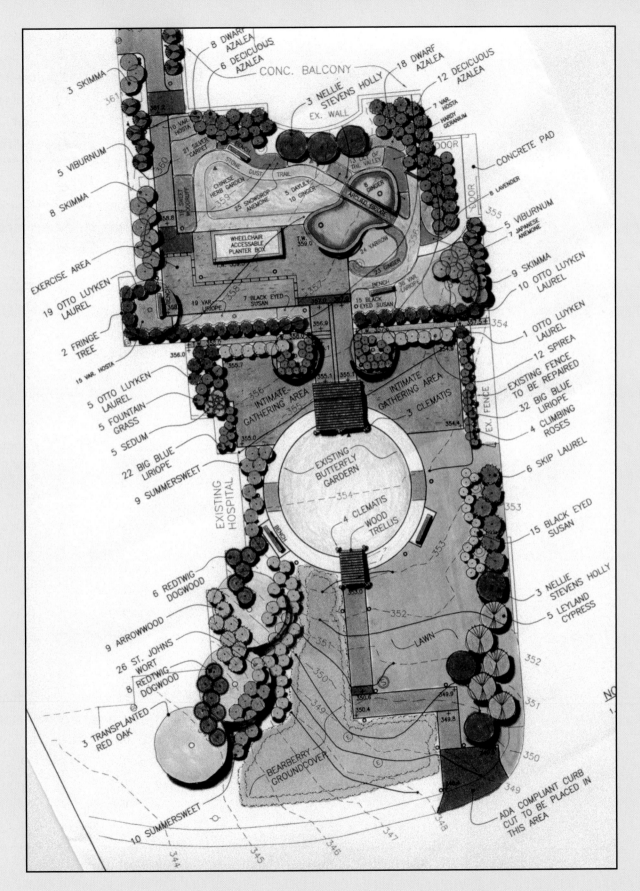

3 SKIMMA

8 DWARF AZALEA

6 DECICUOUS AZALEA

CONC. BALCONY

18 DWARF AZALEA

12 DECICUOUS AZALEA

3 NELLIE STEVENS HOLLY

EX. WALL

7 VAR. HOSTA

HARDY GERANIUM

DOOR

CONCRETE PAD

5 VIBURNUM

10 VAR. HOSTA

21 SILVER CARPET

13 LILY OF THE VALLEY

8 GINGER

DOOR

8 LAVENDER

355

5 VIBURNUM

8 SKIMMA

STONE DUST TRAIL

CHINESE HERB GARDEN

359

25 SNOWDROP ANEMONE

5 DAYLILY

10 GINGER

ARCHED BRIDGE

7 JAPANESE ANEMONE

WOODRUFF

358.8

360

EXERCISE AREA

WHEELCHAIR ACCESSIBLE PLANTER BOX

T.W. 359.0

24 YARROW

23 GINGER

9 SKIMMA

19 OTTO LUYKEN LAUREL

GINGER

360

19 VAR. LIRIOPE

358

7 BLACK EYED SUSAN

38 VAR. LIRIOPE

BENCH

10 OTTO LUYKEN LAUREL

2 FRINGE TREE

357

15 BLACK EYED SUSAN

354

1 OTTO LUYKEN LAUREL

356.9

357.5

15 VAR. HOSTA

356.0

355.7

12 SPIREA

EXISTING FENCE TO BE REPAIRED

5 OTTO LUYKEN LAUREL

INTIMATE GATHERING AREA

INTIMATE GATHERING AREA

32 BIG BLUE LIRIOPE

5 FOUNTAIN GRASS

355.1

355.1

3 CLEMATIS

354.4

4 CLIMBING ROSES

5 SEDUM

355.0

22 BIG BLUE LIRIOPE

6 SKIP LAUREL

EXISTING BUTTERFLY GARDEN

9 SUMMERSWEET

EXISTING HOSPITAL

354

353

BENCH

4 CLEMATIS

WOOD TRELLIS

15 BLACK EYED SUSAN

6 REDTWIG DOGWOOD

353

353.0

3 NELLIE STEVENS HOLLY

9 ARROWWOOD

352

5 LEYLAND CYPRESS

LAWN

26 ST. JOHNS WORT

351

352

8 REDTWIG DOGWOOD

350

349.9

3 TRANSPLANTED RED OAK

349

350.6

349.8

350.4

BEARBERRY GROUNDCOVER

350

349

10 SUMMERSWEET

348

ADA COMPLIANT CURB CUT TO BE PLACED IN THIS AREA

344

345

346

347

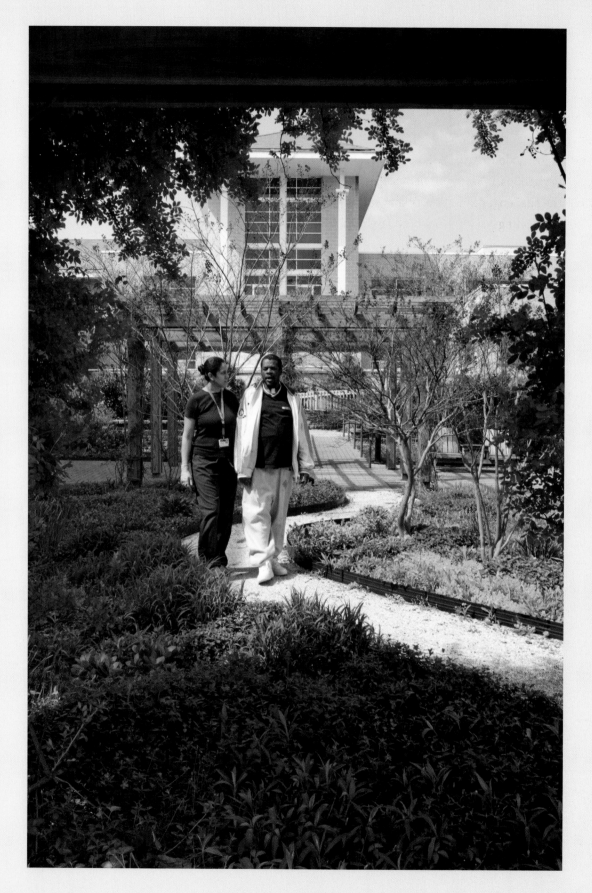

THERAPEUTIC HEALING GARDEN AT KERNAN HOSPITAL

But there was a lot more space on the hospital grounds that could be put to good use. That's when I went back to the TKF Foundation with the idea of a much-expanded rehabilitation garden. They gave us a challenge grant, which again forced us to generate a wide circle of supporters. I created a healing garden advisory board at the hospital, which included people from the community who had different horticultural skills and an interest in gardening. Our CEO became involved, along with the hospital's philanthropy office and a number of community groups. In the end, we raised almost twice as much as we needed to meet the challenge grant. I think that says a lot about the level of support we had for the healing garden, from both the hospital system and the community.

This is also when I started digging in: by reading everything I could get my hands on about healing gardens, by talking to professionals, and by trying to become very clear about what I wanted our garden to look like. I wanted an intimate garden, one that you could get into and feel—as opposed to some of the big, glitzy, upscale designs I had seen. We interviewed four different landscape architecture firms and chose the perfect partner to design our vision. Kernan's healing garden is beautiful, peaceful, and useful, all at the same time.

A healing garden is composed of many different elements. One of them is surfaces and textures. When patients finish their rehabilitation at Kernan, we want to make sure they are safe as they go back into the community. Most of the halls in hospitals have linoleum floors, but that's not what patients are going to have to contend with back in the real world. In creating the garden,

May God bless all who visit this garden and grant them peace. May the Lord bless the doctors and therapists in this hospital for the good work that they do, and may He inspire the nurses and nurses' aides with motivation, compassion, and humility.

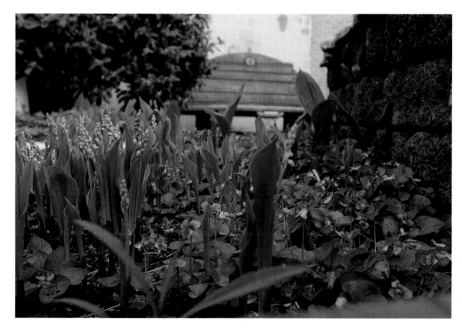

I attempt to share my love for life each and every day by touching people's lives in a positive manner . . . Now I know why I became a nurse. Believe in yourself, have faith, for peace awaits you.

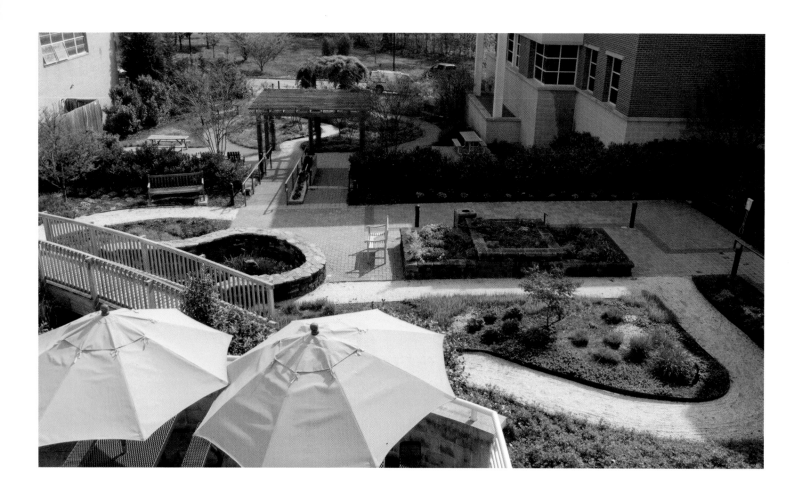

If you can't touch, then smell the flowers.
If you can't smell, then touch the garden.
Don't be down if you've lost something, for
sense all of it with your other abilities.

I wanted to include the variety of textures that patients might have to deal with in the city, in the yard, in the comings and goings of daily life. So we have pavers, cement, grass, and stone dust paths. We have ramps and steps and wooden inclines that cross a bridge. Therapists take patients with varied mobility out to the garden—from patients in wheelchairs to those on crutches to those using walkers or canes to those ambulating on their own. Therapists can take these patients onto different surfaces, to check and see if they are safe. Do they have a bit of a heel drop and difficulty following through with their foot? Do they catch a toe on the pavers or the cobblestones? Do they demonstrate good depth perception when they're going up or down steps? The garden provides a place to identify these kinds of problems and work through them, so that patients have a successful and safe transition back to life outside the hospital.

For people who will continue to be in a wheelchair after they leave the hospital, the garden is designed to be a training course—although you would never know by its appearance. For example, the lily pond and the bridge add great beauty and interest to the garden, but the bridge is also for therapy. It has a slight incline that allows patients to work on wheelchair propulsion. It's more difficult to propel a wheelchair on our stone dust paths than on smoother surfaces, and the patient has to gradually build up strength to be able to do that. The butterfly garden is down toward the bottom of the healing garden, and it's not hard to get to it in a wheelchair. But coming back up again is a whole different story: there is a significant incline that provides another place for strength building. Although many of our patients aren't here long enough to actually get into gardening, we do have wheelchair-height garden beds that have two levels. Patients sitting in wheelchairs can reach into the lower level, and patients working on standing and balancing activities can practice distributing their weight equally on both lower extremities while gardening at the upper level. We also have a lot of adaptive gardening tools that help, like snap-on tool heads that provide extra length for patients who are sitting.

Color is another important element of our healing garden. We wanted plants that would provide colors and textures through all the seasons. At the same time, we wanted our garden to be as eco-friendly as possible, so we took great pains to choose native plants that would meet our color criteria. We have no ground sprinklers in the garden, and even when we recently had a record-breaking drought, most of our plants survived on their own without our watering them—which meant we could spend our time and money in other ways. To keep color and interest in the garden year-round, we chose grasses that keep their plumes into winter: some are red; others are brown. A variety of tree barks provide different colors when the leaves are gone. The red-twig dogwood is lovely in the winter. The holly has berries, and as a result we've had birds nest in the garden. In the spring, summer, and fall, we have practically every color imaginable in the garden. In the butterfly garden, we have Echinacea, butterfly weed, and butterfly bushes, which are all shades of lilac and purple. The crepe myrtle is pink, and the daylilies are orange—butterflies love the oranges and reds. All of this creates a beautiful setting, and it is also part of the rehabilitation process. When a person has a brain injury or stroke, there are cognitive deficits. So we bring these patients out to the garden and ask them to identify things. "Find me something that is yellow," a therapist might say, or "Find me something that smells sweet." We want to see if the patient can follow directions, whether he or she can conceptualize what we're saying verbally and put it into action.

In the summer months, our trellis is covered with the bright magenta flowers of the clematis vine, which is breathtakingly beautiful. But it's there

Warm rays of sunshine
Falling on our faces
Cool breeze in our hair
Love everywhere!

My Daddy moved his finger today.

I have written in here before when I was in this hospital. Now, I'm out. Today the doctor told me I can start walking. I can't believe it. I really can't. Now, I can make footprints.

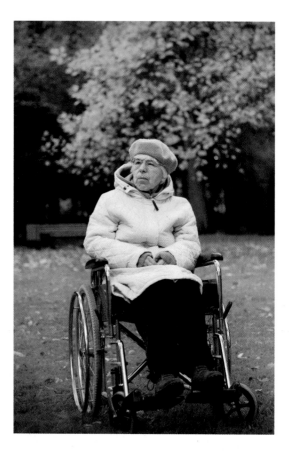

for another reason—to provide shade, which is extremely important for some of our patients. After a spinal cord injury, particularly in our quadriplegic patients, the body doesn't have the ability to regulate its temperature. These patients are essentially in a new body that they are still in the process of getting to know. Temperature is a nuance that they can easily forget, which could lead to sunburn or heat stroke, so we wanted to create spaces for them to get out of the sun. These shady areas also provide space for more private interactions, whether a speech therapist working with a patient on oral motor articulation skills or a conversation between a family and a patient. Like everything else in the garden, benches have more than one purpose. They are there to provide places for people to sit and enjoy the peace of the garden. But equally important, the benches keep our patients safe by providing resting places for them, as they meet new and harder challenges in their therapy.

Beauty is an essential element of our healing garden too, not just an extra frill but part of the healing process. A study has been done that compared two groups of hospital patients. They both had the same kind of health issues and the same procedure, but one group of people looked out of their hospital windows at a brick wall, while the other group looked out at trees. The people who looked at trees used less pain medication, felt less stress, and had lower blood pressure. This isn't surprising to me. It just confirms what my own experience with gardening has taught me—that gardens help keep people healthy by allowing them to be outdoors and by giving them a way to relax and de-stress. And the garden works not only for the healing of our patients but for others as well. Staff members use the garden in between shift changes, as a way to collect themselves if they are having a difficult day, or just as a quiet place for lunch outside of the hospital. Having a place to escape for a short time from a computer screen or the walls of an office or the halls of the hospital can make a big difference in the overall well-being of the staff. In addition, the families of our patients are often under a lot of stress, and the garden provides a peaceful place for them to meet with their loved ones or just have a quiet moment alone.

We haven't done any formal research to measure the healing effects of the garden. But if you measure results based on the use of the garden, it is a success. And based on the journal entries, people are certainly grateful. One patient, reflecting on what he had been through and what lay ahead for him, said, "This garden gives me a sense that there is still a God." Another wrote, "Today I rolled my wheelchair across the stone dust path; someday I hope to walk across it." Others have told us, "This garden is wonderful. It allowed me to visit with my family." Patients have written thank-you letters to the hospital for the garden. One woman was so grateful for what we had done for her son that every year after he had left, she donated herbs for our wheelchair-height garden. Then she had an herb sale in her town and sent the proceeds to us to use for the healing garden.

One patient in particular stands out in my mind—a man who had a motorcycle accident and came to us with so many broken bones it was hard to count them, and fingers that were completely smashed. He loves gardening, and he used it as therapy to work on both standing activities to strengthen his legs, which have steel rods in them, and activities to improve the manipulation of his hands. He then went on to teach himself quill art as another activity to keep his hands moving—and he got so good at it that the cards he makes have been sold at the Baltimore Museum of Art. He is so grateful to be able to do something he loves that he comes back every now and then to teach our patients quill art, and he always goes out to spend some time in the garden. This is what our healing garden is all about—getting our patients to the point where they can do the things they love and feel good about themselves. When I witness stories like this, and there are many, I know the garden is doing its work. My dream is to see healing gardens like ours at hospitals all across the country.

To the ones who need comfort from their grief or their loss: I hope you find comfort in these pages, this place, this moment.

Dear Lord,
Thank you for watching out over my Dad and giving him the courage to try to get better . . . I pray for strength for all of us, including my Mom.

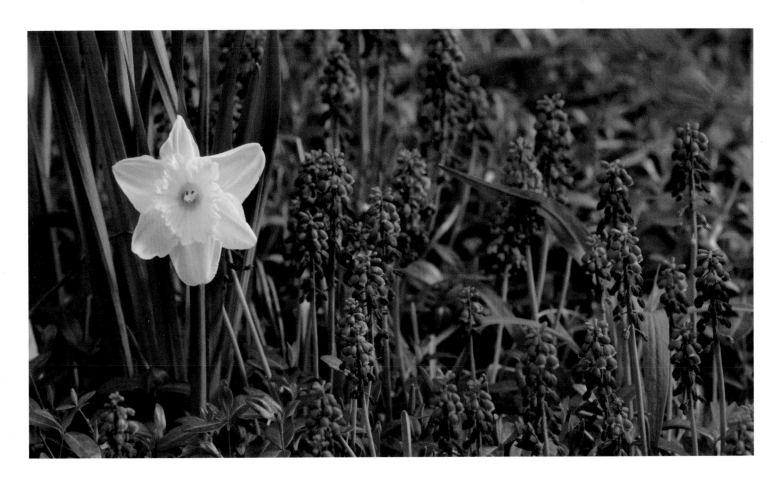

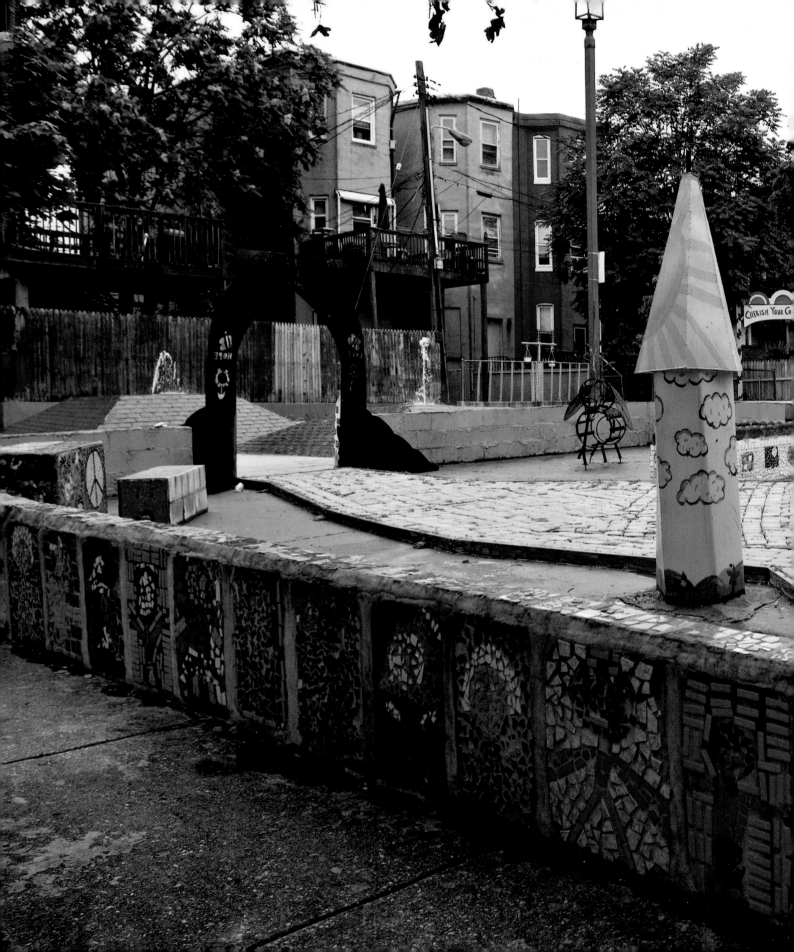

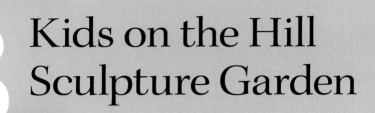

8 Kids on the Hill Sculpture Garden

It's not rocket science to get the kids on your side. You have to make them feel a part of the community rather than apart from the community.

— Rebecca Yenawine, Firesoul

Like so many inner city neighborhoods in America, the area that surrounds Reservoir Hill in Baltimore City is deeply challenged. Despite many caring and dedicated residents, there are abandoned lots and abandoned homes, an active drug trade, a struggling school, no supermarket, and no economic infrastructure—leaving residents without essential resources.

Growing up in a lower income neighborhood can have a devastating impact on youth. These children face challenges that many people could never even imagine. They are forced to take on responsibilities that are beyond their capacity to fulfill. Their childhood is too quickly sacrificed, replaced by the struggle to survive. When youth and creativity are robbed, something very valuable gets lost along the way: confidence, goals for the future, and hope that one's life could make a difference. Many young people, under this pressure, can become a source of crime in their own communities.

Rebecca Yenawine moved to Reservoir Hill in 1991 to study art at a nearby college, but the native New Yorker quickly learned that the true classroom was in her backyard. She focused her attention on the kids, determined to

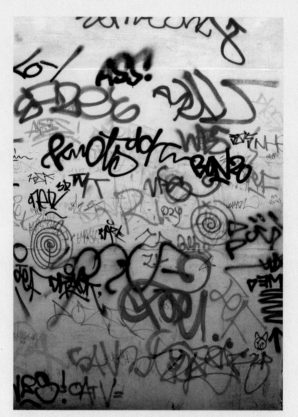

use the arts to help them combat stereotypes and discouragement. Using her skills as an artist and listener, she helped to bring out the creativity and insights of the young people. Through art, they grappled with disruptive forces and transformed the issues into something uplifting and hopeful. As a result, the kids began to see the possibility of a better community for themselves. With Rebecca's guidance, the kids created a very special sculpture garden that is now an oasis in the neighborhood. Through nurturing the young people's creativity, Rebecca helped them become part of the solution. As new neighbors moved in and became invested in the community, they saw the role that young people could have in revitalization, and they in turn were inspired.

Rebecca had no map, no institutional plan in place to help her accomplish this vision. She had only her belief that art and imagination could transform a disconnected community into a unified one, through the creation of a laboratory for creative expression. She and the kids turned an abandoned lot into a place for all to experience and enjoy. Woven in with the Kids on the Hill sculpture park is a small garden area with a bench and a journal, so that nature also plays a part in the healing. This project brings the best part of human nature together with nature itself. Rebecca then convinced the City of Baltimore to partner with her organization. This valuable step gave an added sense of permanence and empowerment to the budding enterprise. Adults and youth together have contributed to a sculpture park that depicts their dreams for a better life and a better neighborhood. Together they converted a place of turmoil into a space of safety and sacredness.

Today, Rebecca and her co-director, Mark Carter, have a plan for making neighborhood changes happen. They use the idea of "art for social change" as their motto and have set in motion another valuable legacy: they have inspired young teachers to join in, like sculptor Jesse Reid. Rebecca's combination of creative and entrepreneurial skills along with the dedication of her neighbors and the young people themselves ensure that the Kids on the Hill sculpture garden can remain a viable and valuable part of this community for years to come.

—*T.S.*

Rebecca Yenawine

Co-Director and Artistic Director, Kids on the Hill Inc.

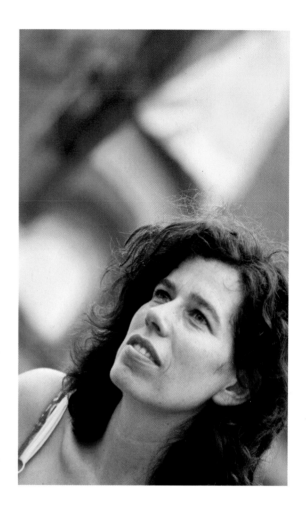

I fell in love with Reservoir Hill in 1991, when I was going to art school nearby, and I rented an apartment here. My childhood in New York City was privileged, and as a result, I have sought out the experience of being a minority in a community. It forces me to think about myself and my identity as a white person, and I like what I learn from being with people who are different from me.

I was studying at the Maryland Institute College of Art, but I dropped out after about a year and a half. It was during the Persian Gulf War, and I expected that my fellow artists would have a response to the war. In my mind, art and social action go hand in hand. I consider artists to be truth-sayers and visionaries, people who can imagine a much more elegant solution than war. But I found that very few of my classmates cared. I also believe that art should be active and inclusive, and I wasn't finding my path in the systems that were set up for artists at the school. At the same time, I knew that I was committed to art. I also knew that I didn't want to leave the neighborhood. So I bought a house about a block away that was incredibly inexpensive. And there I was—a homeowner in my early twenties!

I got to know the children in the neighborhood by working in my backyard. I could hear them in the alley, and I would go out and introduce myself. Eventually, they started coming over to visit, and I began carving out time in my day to spend with them. We would play piano, make apple juice, draw—whatever I was doing, they would join in. Then one day, I caught three teenage girls spray painting. I took their paint and invited them in for an art lesson. They loved it and came back week after week, studying figure drawing and painting, and eventually painting their self-portraits. They got permission from a landlord and the neighborhood association to paint over the boarded windows and doors of three abandoned buildings. Less than six months after I caught them spray painting, their portraits and other art covered nine windows and doors and brightened the whole block. The girls were proud of their art, and when the younger children walked by, they felt proud of their older friends. Instead of seeing graffiti and the negative statement it sometimes makes, adults saw how creative and talented the neighborhood teens were. This was the first time I was able to see how art had the possibility for changing a group of young people—and possibly even a community.

At this point, my projects with the kids had outgrown my house, so we found another location to meet. I started raising money for an after-school program, which became Kids on the Hill Inc. in 1997. I think that *after-school program* often conjures up a vision of a lot of kids chasing a basketball around a gymnasium. I'm not saying that isn't a valuable thing to do, but our program is different. It's an art and media program that focuses on social justice. We provide young people with higher level skill-building opportunities so that they can become media-makers, artists, good citizens, and competent leaders.

In 1999, with funding from the TKF Foundation, we started to create a sculpture garden, which was a project of our first summer camp. The site where the garden now stands was a vacant park that was nothing more than a big piece of concrete with broken glass scattered across it. It had become an open-air drug market, with neighbors complaining about the drug activity and about people getting drunk and being noisy late at night.

We began our garden project by focusing on the theme of castles. Every child knows that castles are where kings, queens, princes, and princesses live, and they are powerful people. So we set out to create a castle in our neighborhood where youth could be powerful. At the same time, we gave them a way to address issues of power and class. We asked the children, "If you were

Places like this make me feel like everything will be OK.

The park is nice because it looks like fun for a picnic

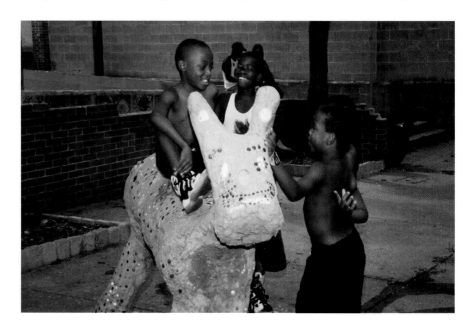

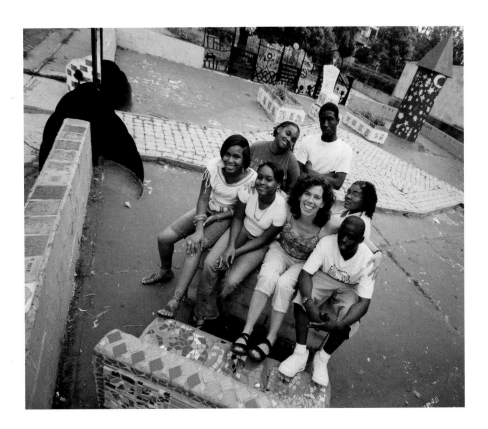

king or queen, what would you change about your world to make it better?" The answers to that question are embedded in the sculptures in the garden:

"If I were king for a day, I would make a type of skin lotion so everyone would have the same skin color, so no one could be racist."

"If I were queen, I would give all the poor people money and toys."

Every project we do has three parts. First, we study. The children learned about castles, they looked at pictures, and they figured out what imagery appealed to them. The second phase was for them to design the imagery they wanted in the garden. For example, they wanted a tower, so each child drew a picture of a tower, and the group voted on the one they liked best. Then, finally, the children brought their images into reality. They created three welded metal towers, a mosaic throne, a mosaic table and benches for games and picnics, numerous images, and a wall of tiles that surrounds the garden. The words of the children are included as well, expressing their visions for a better world.

The towers are big—one is nine feet tall—so we're talking about an ambitious project! We had artists working with and teaching the children all summer long—a mosaic artist, a casting artist, and a welding artist. Learning how to use power tools was a very empowering experience for the

We saw a bird that we tried to catch. A fun place to dig with sticks, looking for worms. We came here to see other people in the neighborhood.

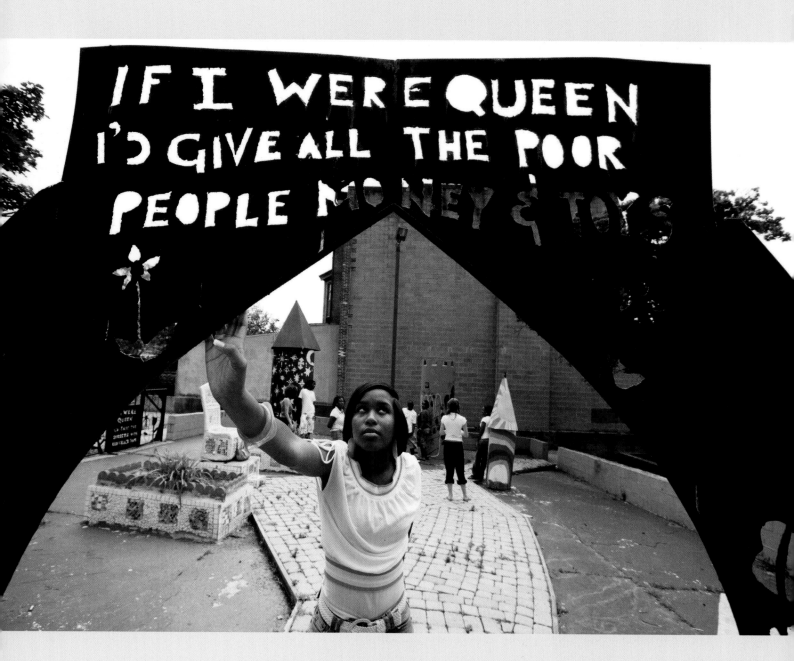

young people, especially for the girls. They used circular saws, jigsaws, plasma cutters, and welding electric grinders. To see one of the "girliest" girls wearing a welding hat and feeling comfortable with getting dirty was exciting for me. The project built self-confidence in every one of the children who worked on it.

But it empowered them in another way too. Their art is visible in their community, and therefore they are visible. Every time they walk by the garden, they get to say, "I made that. That's my piece right there. That was my idea." They also get to see other people, both youth and adults, interact with their art, and that enhances their sense of self. The garden gives young people a voice in their neighborhood, a way to be seen and heard, a way to have ownership in their community.

You can see that ownership in the way they take care of the garden. Often, when adults think of what young people can do for their community, they ask them to come out for a cleanup day. In my experience, that's not really what young people enjoy. But I've noticed that when they pick up trash in their sculpture garden, it's a very different experience. It doesn't feel to them like they are being used to pick up somebody else's junk. It feels more like they are cleaning up their own rooms, and they get to enjoy and appreciate their artwork. There's no dignity in picking up someone else's trash, but keeping the sculpture garden clean has a lot of dignity, because it's theirs.

Another thing that has strengthened their connection to each other, and therefore strengthened the community, is the teamwork they've learned from creating the sculpture garden together. Whether it's drawing designs, learning to use a tape measure, marking, cutting, or welding, we break the tasks down as much as possible, so that each person knows what he or she is contributing to the group and how that group is contributing to the final goal. It is always a group effort, a collaboration, to get a project created and finished.

In the eight years since we began the sculpture garden—and it remains an ongoing project—its young creators have witnessed the impact that their work has had on the community. Each year we have a festival in the park. One of the neighbors is our grill-master. We count on him to bring out his giant grill and cook up hamburgers and hot dogs. Another neighbor is a musician, and he puts up his huge speakers so that people can hear his music all over the neighborhood. I truly feel transported when we have our summer festivals, as if I'm in a different world.

On summer evenings, people bring folding chairs and sit and watch movies shown on a screen hung from the stage we designed in a corner of the park. There is also a fountain. Playing in it provides the children endless entertainment. In another part of the park, there is a lovely bench from TFK, which people use to read or meditate. All around it are flowers, many of them

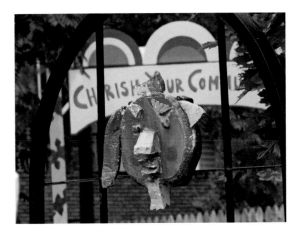

Beauty is a child's imagination in practice.

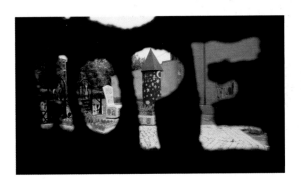

I am remembering Jason who died long ago, at age 15 because he didn't know he was loved, wanted, and valued. May he rest in peace, and may we all learn to cherish our children.

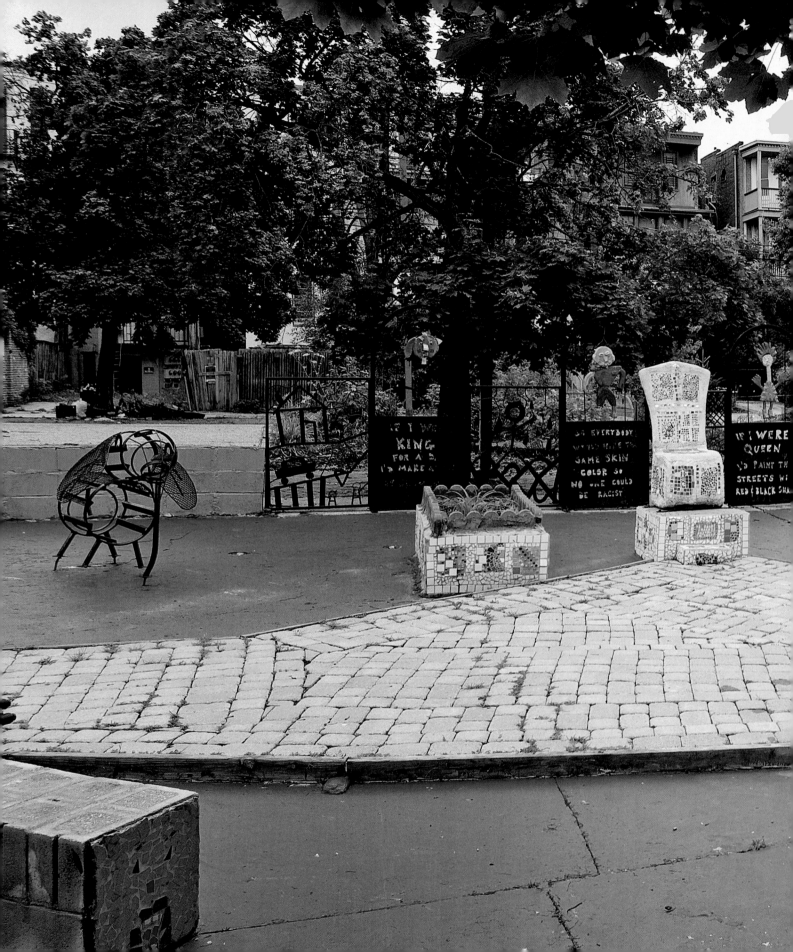

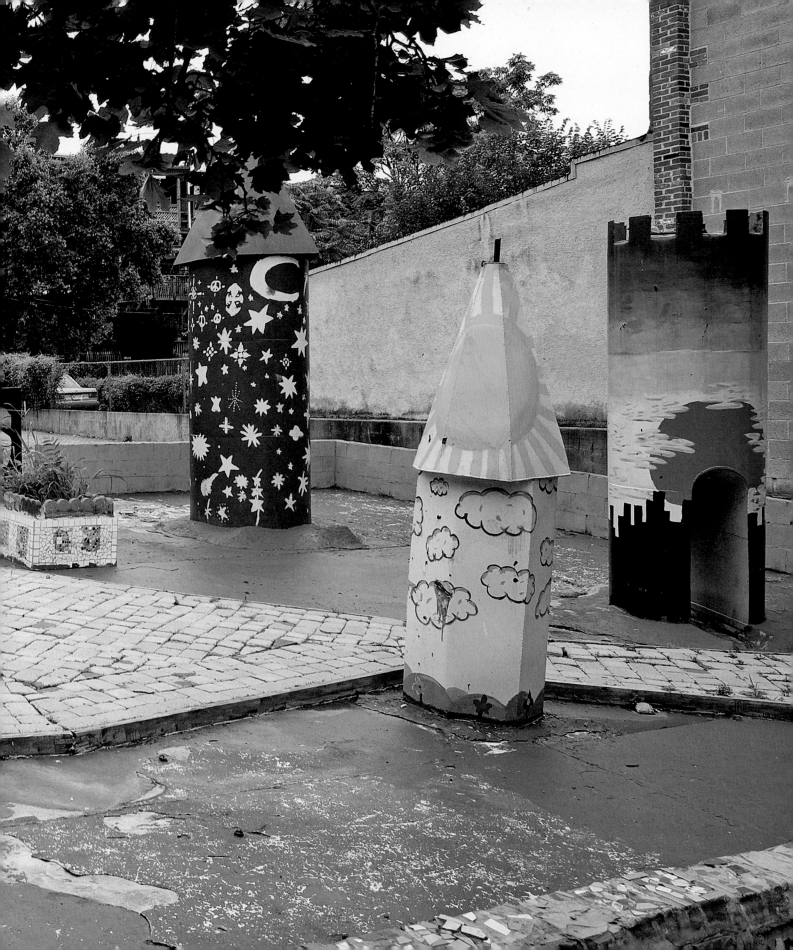

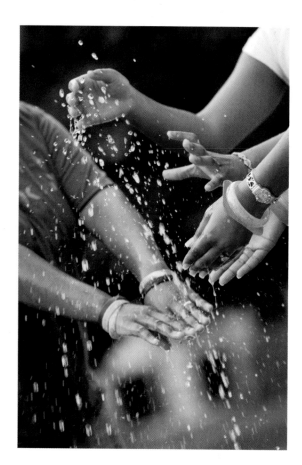

This is a reservoir of peace in a busy world. It gives one the possibility to hear the spirit within.

planted by a neighbor. She said her yard just wasn't big enough for all the flowers she wanted to grow, and she asked if she could extend her garden to the park. Now she and the Kids on the Hill children tend the flowers together.

Not all of the activities are planned. Recently, the neighborhood had a cleanup day and afterward, people spontaneously came to the park to grill and picnic and talk together. The sculpture garden—the vision and the work of the neighborhood children—serves as the center of what has become an important and vibrant community gathering place. This place that was once a drug hangout is now used by neighbors of all ages; and lots of people, young and old, consider themselves guardians of the space.

I always learn as much from young people as they do from me, and one of the things I've learned from creating this sculpture garden with them is how powerful it is for a community to have a youth space. In communities that are newer and more middle class, they plan for children to have play space. I think it's absolutely vital to provide that same thing in older communities as well. Young people have an incredible amount to contribute to community issues. If they aren't engaged in some way in the life of the community, they won't be on the community's side, the side of making a positive difference. It's not rocket science to get the kids on your side, and it's not rocket science to figure out what leads them to be vandals. You have to make them feel *a part of* the community rather than *apart from* the community.

There's no end of ideas that we can come up with to add to the sculpture garden. Each year, we have initiated a new project to involve more children. So far, more than a hundred children have contributed to the garden. This is vital to creating an ongoing sense of ownership that will make younger children want to be the guardians of the art of those who came before them. But as the years pass, we also have to focus on repairing and maintaining what we already have, so that people continue to respect it. At this point, we must balance the two.

Fortunately, Kids on the Hill continues to attract other staff members like Jesse Reid, who are as passionately dedicated to sculpture instruction and the garden as I am. Ironically, Jesse found his way to Kids on the Hill through an internship with the Maryland Institute College of Art. He was earning his master's degree in their Art and Community Arts program—the kind of program I wanted sixteen years ago but wasn't available—and the sculpture garden attracted him. What a blessing he's been! Watching Jesse's commitment to the garden grow and deepen over the year we've worked together has taught me something very important about sacred places—no one person owns them. You put the torch into the hands of the next Firesoul and pass it on.

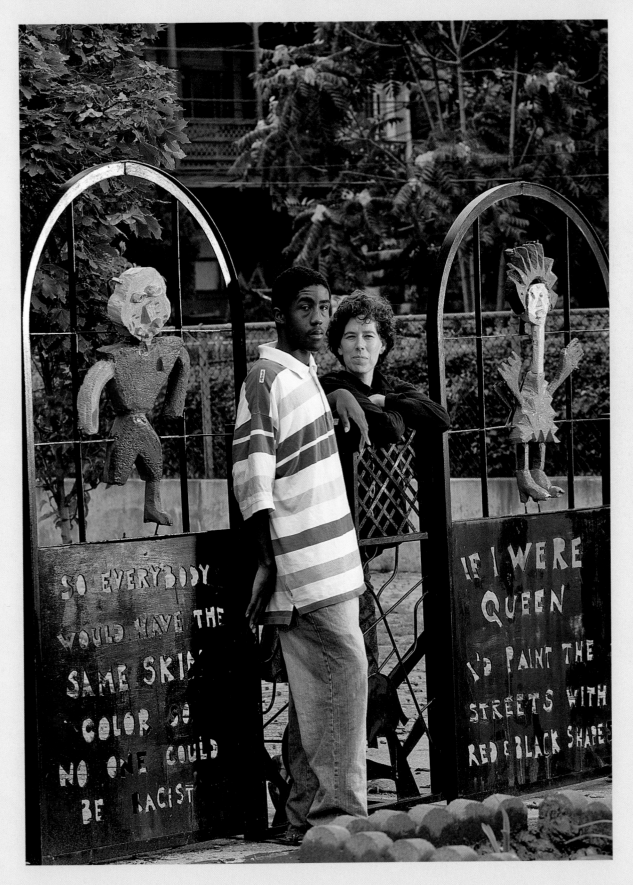

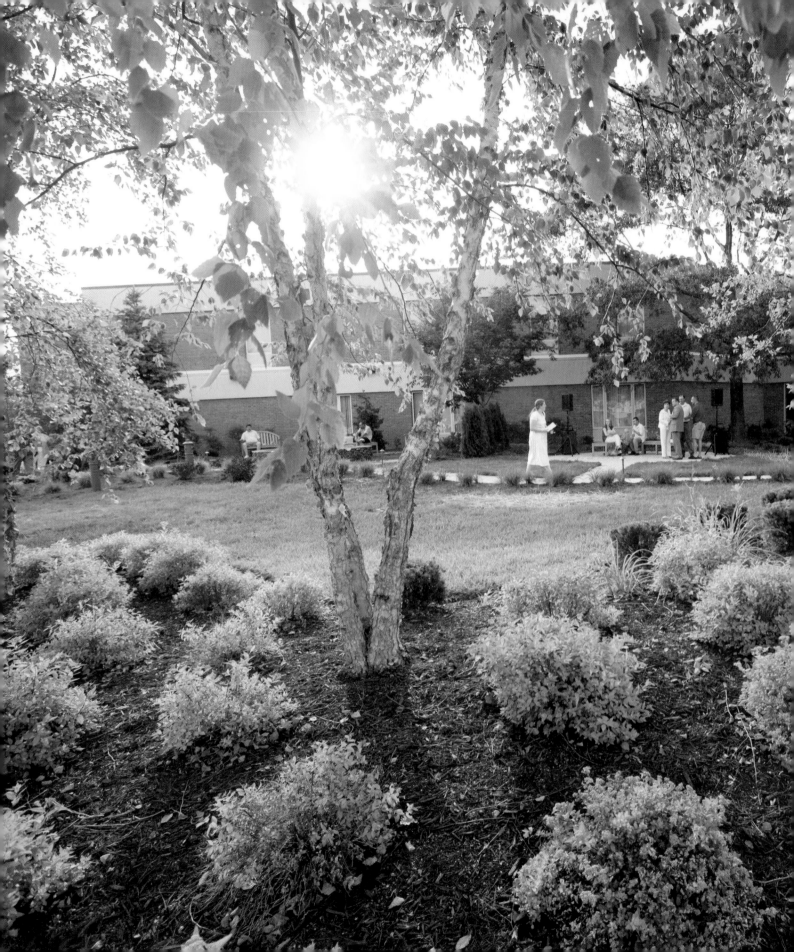

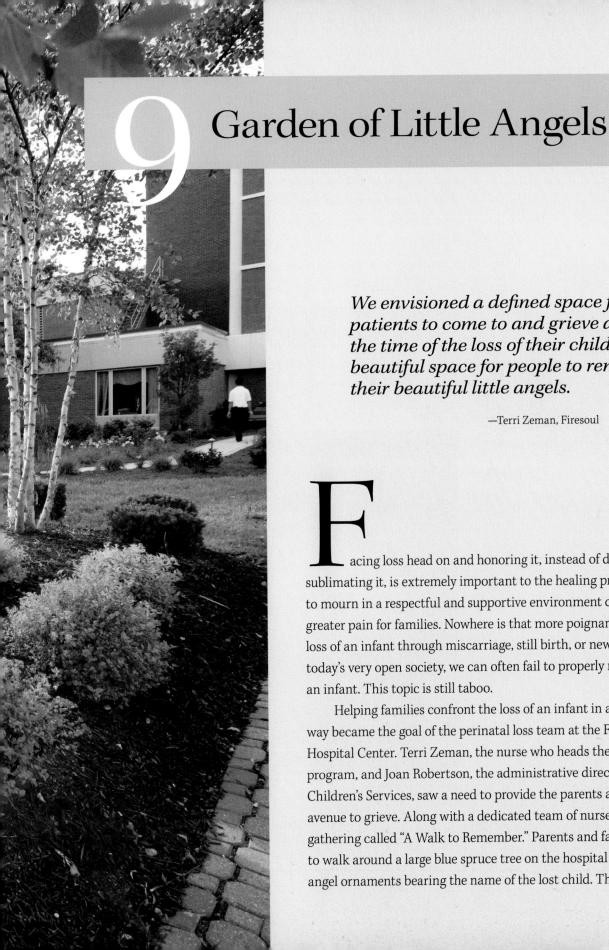

9 Garden of Little Angels

We envisioned a defined space for patients to come to and grieve at the time of the loss of their child. A beautiful space for people to remember their beautiful little angels.

—Terri Zeman, Firesoul

Facing loss head on and honoring it, instead of denying or sublimating it, is extremely important to the healing process. The inability to mourn in a respectful and supportive environment can often lead to even greater pain for families. Nowhere is that more poignantly felt than in the loss of an infant through miscarriage, still birth, or newborn death. Even in today's very open society, we can often fail to properly recognize the loss of an infant. This topic is still taboo.

Helping families confront the loss of an infant in an honest and caring way became the goal of the perinatal loss team at the Franklin Square Hospital Center. Terri Zeman, the nurse who heads the perinatal loss program, and Joan Robertson, the administrative director for Women's and Children's Services, saw a need to provide the parents and families with an avenue to grieve. Along with a dedicated team of nurses, they began with a gathering called "A Walk to Remember." Parents and families were invited to walk around a large blue spruce tree on the hospital grounds and to hang angel ornaments bearing the name of the lost child. That tree became the

Find Peace within yourself
Treat others the way you want to be
   treated
Smile and be happy for the simple
   things
Be happy to be able to see, walk,
   breathe
And to be able to enjoy the
Open space, sacred place
That surrounds you

center of an annual ceremony that grew over ten years. The nurses began to see the need for a bigger, more defined garden of healing, one centered around that tree, that would include components to help every family member—mother, father, sibling, relative—find peace.

As you might imagine, a hospital can struggle with where to put its financial resources to use. Administrative decisions often lean toward investing in infrastructures that prevent death, like a new cancer wing. A very valuable lesson that we have learned over the years from our Firesouls is the importance of perseverance. Without it, none of the projects highlighted in this book would have come to fruition. That trait is perhaps most vividly shown in this story—of how the nurses at Franklin Square, after many, many years, finally built their Garden of Little Angels. Today, this garden is a permanent and valuable part of Franklin Square, and it is a space that supplies lasting support to bereaved families.

—*T.S.*

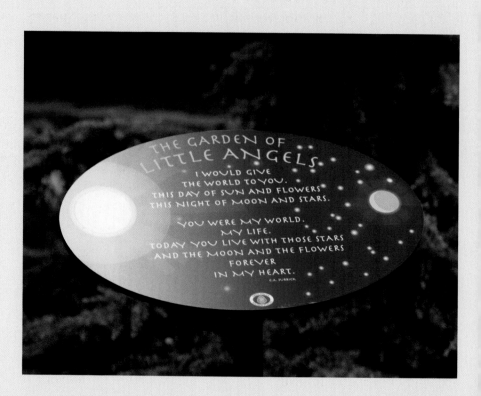

Terri Zeman, RN

Perinatal Loss Program Coordinator, Franklin Square Hospital Center

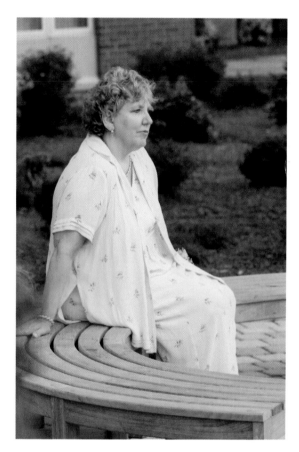

Most people think of Labor and Delivery as a happy place in a hospital, and most of the time it is. But when it's sad, it's really sad. Of the thousands of births at our hospital each year, about forty families experience the loss of a baby—through miscarriage, stillbirth, or newborn death. It's devastating, because they not only lose the baby; they lose their dreams and hopes for the child's future. What happens at that terrible moment—the kind of support the parents get or don't get from the hospital staff—can make all the difference in the world. In 1988, Franklin Square Hospital began a focused effort to better meet the needs of our patients in that situation.

At that time, I was part of a group that created specific guidelines for how to care for the patient experiencing a perinatal loss. People have a hard time discussing the death of a baby. In the past, the grieving part of the experience was often swept under the rug. But the general thinking was changing—moving toward more discussing what had happened, more holding of the baby, and more acknowledging the baby's life, however brief. Our guidelines included an educational program for nurses, physicians, and hospital staff, to improve their ability to respond in a helpful way to patients who are experiencing a loss. Then in 1992, I saw a real need for an ongoing support group for parents who had lost their babies. I started HUGS—"Healing and Understanding through Group Support." The group meets once a month and welcomes patients from our hospital as well as from other area hospitals.

We then created "A Walk to Remember," a yearly gathering at the hospital on the first weekend of November, to which we invite all those who have experienced a loss, along with any guests they want to bring. We walk around a large blue spruce tree on which people hang angel ornaments bearing the

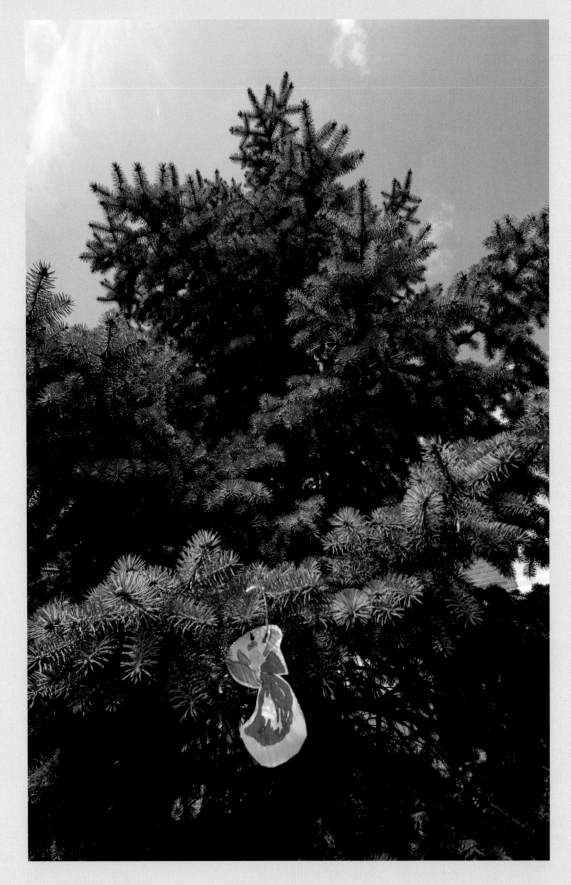

name of the child they lost. This simple act gradually evolved into a service with music and poetry and time for parents and families to talk with each other. For babies who were cremated by the hospital, there is no gravesite: this is the only place parents can come to remember their child. For many, this is a very important opportunity to be with others who have experienced a similar loss and to get support from those who truly understand.

A couple of years after we began "A Walk to Remember," some of the nurses—and also some of the parents—began to think how nice it would be to have a garden in the area surrounding the spruce tree. We began to dream. We envisioned a defined space for parents to grieve at the time of the loss of their child. A beautiful space for people to remember their beautiful "little angels." A sacred space to honor death and life, to be sorrow-filled and to celebrate. That's how the idea for our Garden of Little Angels was born, and it was then, about ten years ago, that the nurses of the perinatal loss team began to raise funds to make it happen.

Despite our enthusiasm, despite the countless hours we spent on bake sales, raffles, and other events—despite the total commitment of Paula Fiorucci, Grace Bourke, Janice Colbert, and Kellie Zink to raise the funds to make our dream a reality—it became apparent that we would never raise enough money on our own to create the garden. We had the unwavering support of Joan Robertson, the administrative director for Women's and Children's Services. As the voice for the nurses on the unit, Joan kept putting the idea of the garden in front of the administration; she simply did not give up. But as in most medical institutions, there were many concerns vying for limited dollars. At the same time, a new hospital building was constructed, so the garden ended up at the bottom of the priority list. We began to talk about another way of raising the money. That's when we found TKF, whose support enabled us to add the final piece to what I consider a world-class perinatal loss program.

One of the hardest things about a perinatal loss is the lack of tangible memories from the child's life. If parents lose a child who is older, they have photos, toys, and clothing they can keep to remember the child. But there is very little that the mother experiencing a perinatal loss can hold in her hand and say, "Yes, I was a mother. I am a mother." I believe that one of the roles of health-care professionals in helping parents whose babies have died is to make the experience real. That was one of the strong motivations for creating a remembrance garden—a physical place that is always there as witness to the baby's life, however short it was.

One way to help make the experience real, a way we've been using for years, is to create a memory box for the parents. The box contains as many

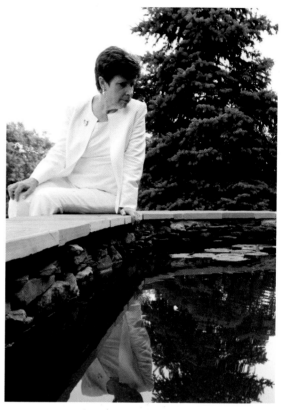

Joan Robertson, Firesoul

The peace and beauty of this garden help heal the hurts and pain and make the world seem whole again.

Thank you for sending me angels to guide me in my journey.

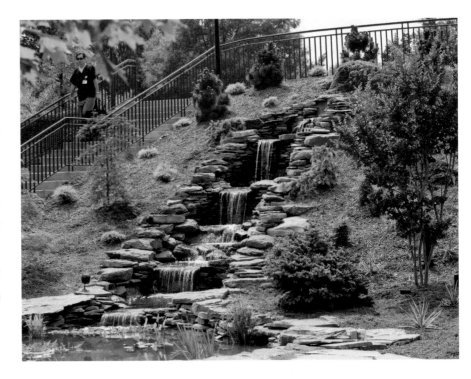

من مادرم حدود 3 ماه پیش مریض بود و مریضی خطرناکی بود.

خدا کمک ما کرد و مادرم خوب شد. من خدا را شکر میکنم.

من 1 دختر 11 ساله هستم

روحیه

I have come to the garden today in honor of what would be William's 13th birthday. As you rest in heaven today and days to come, I sit and cry because I miss you so very much. I wish Daddy and I were able to be with you longer, enjoy you for who you would be. It hurts so much every day to miss, love, and want you to be a part of our life. As I sit and cry, I wonder what you would like, who you would look like, and what you would be doing. We miss you . . . Happy birthday, William. Love, Mom and Dad

mementos as possible of the baby. If the parent agrees, we take a photo of the baby. We usually also put into the box a newborn cap, a small blanket, an armband, a locket of hair if possible, handprints, and footprints. This is all done with the permission of the parents. We do have some parents who don't want a memory box or whose cultures don't condone it, and we're always respectful of that. After the parents go home, we send them a sympathy card signed by the nurse who did the delivery, on behalf of the nursing and medical staff.

We encourage the parents to hold the baby, and we stress that this is the only chance they will have to do this. When the death is sudden and unexpected, the parents are often completely disoriented. They look to the nurses and doctors to help guide them in what to do. I usually tell the parents what other parents have found beneficial. I even encourage them to imagine it's a year later, that they're looking back on this event, and I ask them what they wish they had done or not done. In all my years, I have never had a family say, "I wish we hadn't photographed the baby." But they have said, "I wish we had loved the baby more, kissed the baby more, let other family members see the baby."

People grieve in different ways. With the loss of a baby, the parents often experience something called *disenfranchised grief* or *silent grief*. It occurs when the parents' grief isn't supported by family and friends. People mistakenly

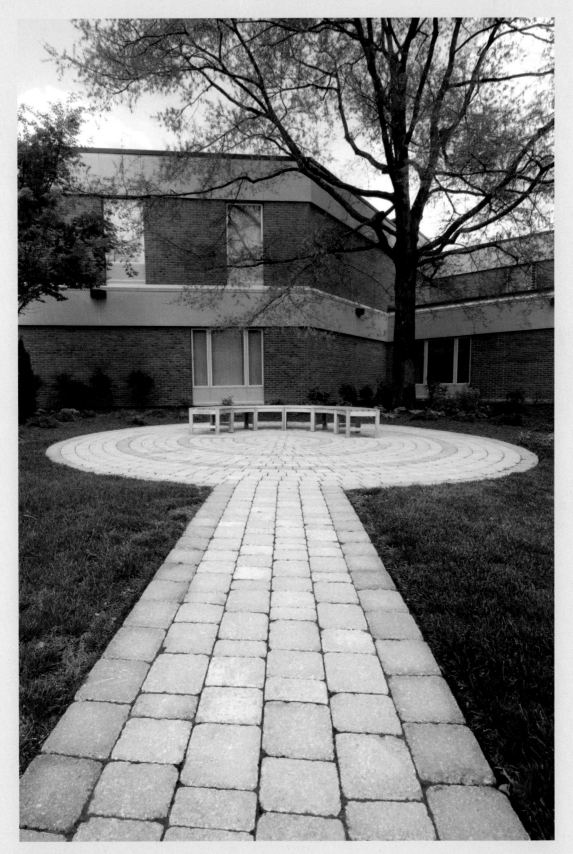

Path to children's labyrinth

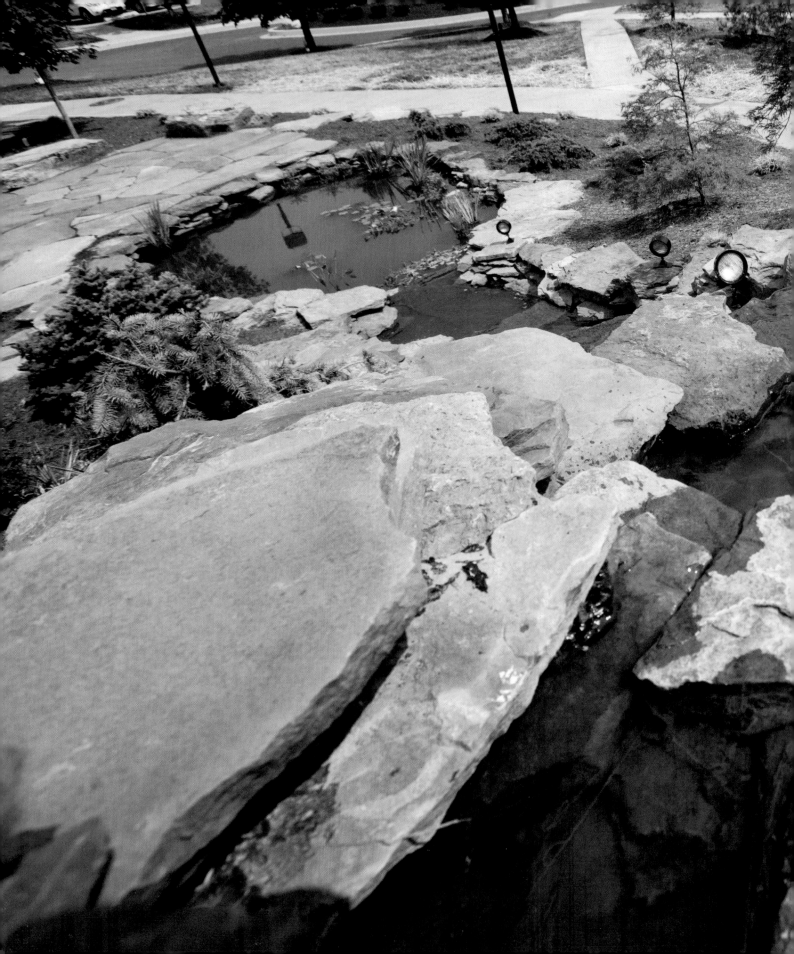

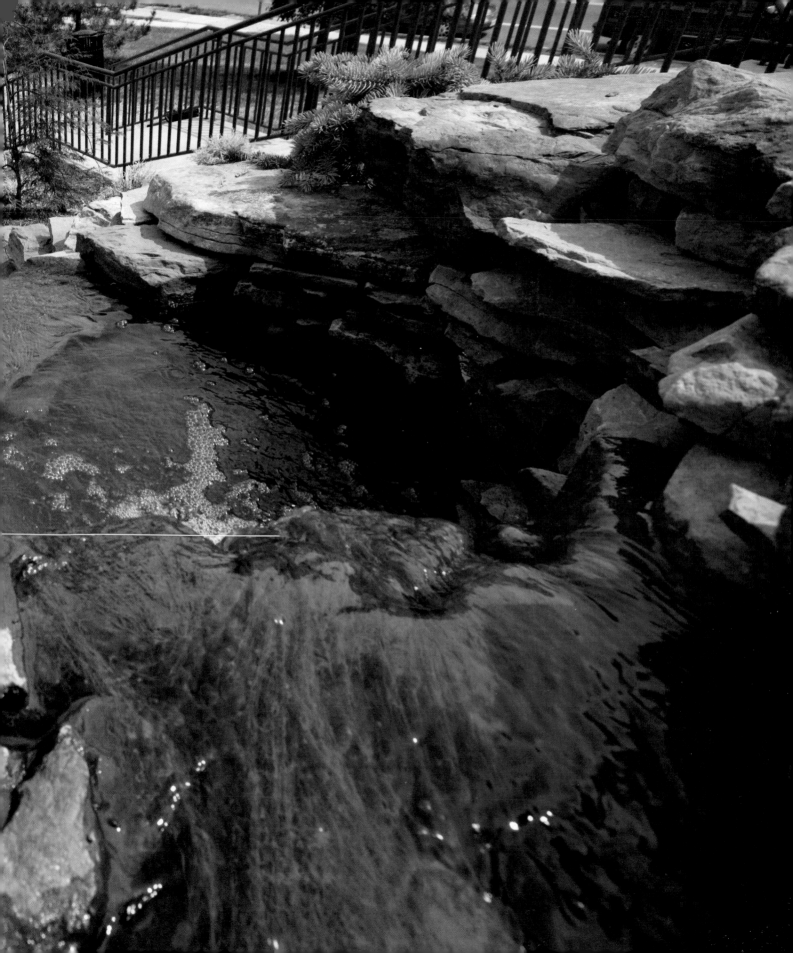

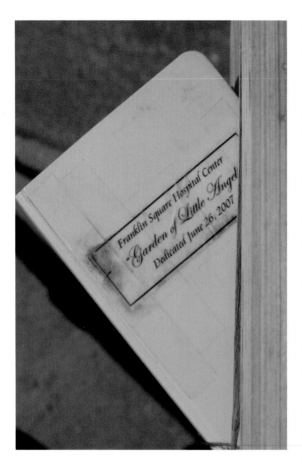

think that because the baby died in the womb or right after birth, there isn't really a life to grieve. Because no one else acknowledges the loss, these parents may suffer in silence.

We think that acknowledgment should begin right away in the hospital, so we educate everyone who works in the department. For example, it's terrible if someone from the housekeeping staff walks into a room where the parents have experienced a loss and says, "Oh, what did you have: a boy or a girl?" We put a teardrop on the door so that all the hospital staff—from nurses to housekeepers to dietary aides—will be aware of the loss. We also realize that it can present an uncomfortable situation, so we educate our staff to say something like, "Mrs. So-and-So, I'm really sorry to hear about your loss." Something as little as that empowers our staff to be helpful, and it is tremendously powerful to the family to hear the loss articulated.

It's important to remember that the size of the baby has nothing to do with the gravity or length of the grief experienced by the parents. It's also interesting to see what can happen when the grief is acknowledged. I had a couple in HUGS that was having a very, very hard time dealing with the death of their baby. When it came time for our yearly memorial service, I reminded them that they could bring friends and family with them. They brought eight or nine people. At the next HUGS meeting, the father said, "You know, my family just didn't get it until they came to the service and saw all the sadness." Then he said, "You know what my mom did? When she renewed her driver's

This beautiful little book has helped me cry and helped me heal . . . I sat down in the shadow, and now I am in the light of the sun—and your love, but I know it was always so.

The cool breezes blow against my tear-shed face, and my eyes will soon close. I shall let the sounds of the waterfall fill my soul, the bright color of spring blooms chase away my blues for just a little while.

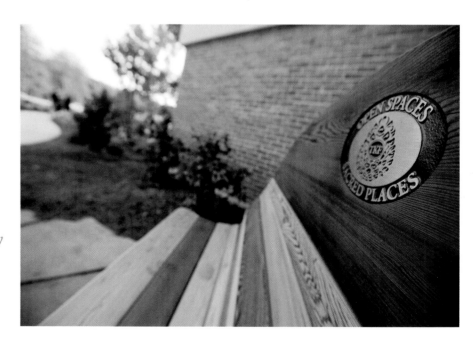

license, she had the baby's name put on the tag." The experience wasn't real for the couple until those to whom they were closest acknowledged the baby's life and death. Then the healing began for real.

Sometimes the couple doesn't really grieve the loss of a baby until a healthy child is born. Then the parent begins to wonder, "What did I miss with John?" or "What would Emily look like now?" As a nurse, I can be more sensitive to the parents if I know that there was a loss prior to the delivery: the experience of delivering a healthy baby after a loss can be bittersweet.

Then there are the brothers and sisters of the baby who dies. Just like their parents, they have been anticipating the arrival of a new little person in the house, and now there is no one to bring home from the hospital. Sometimes the parents are torn on whether to let other children view the baby brother or sister. I counsel the parents to let each child make his or her own decision if the child is old enough, say three or four. Sometimes an older child will help me bathe the baby and dress it before the baby is taken down to the morgue—a sort of symbolic putting the baby to bed.

Our Garden of Little Angels is a soothing place for parents and siblings to sort through their feelings. Nestled against the walls of the Women's Pavilion, the garden includes a thirty-foot-tall waterfall, meandering walkways, a pond filled with lily pads, and a number of quiet spaces for reflection. It has a children's area, with a miniature labyrinth where children can walk or run in circles to their hearts' content and have the space they need at this difficult time. Central to the garden is the blue spruce tree that is the focus of our annual ceremony honoring the lost babies.

I'm very proud of our perinatal loss program and of all we've done over the years to keep building it to meet the needs of grieving parents. And now our garden is the icing on the cake—a physical place, a sacred space where families can grieve the loss and celebrate the life. The fact is, our hospital has an outstanding women's program. We deliver 2,600 healthy babies every year. But we also have about forty families who need something different from us. Now, because of the perseverance of a few dedicated people, we can offer those families the very best support. It's been a long hard road, but worth every step.

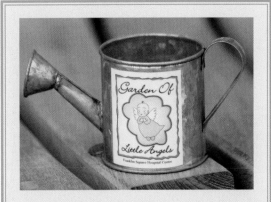

I MYSELF EXPERIENCED A LOSS thirty years ago when I delivered at Franklin Square, and my baby died. That was in the days when the hospital staff really didn't do anything for the parents in such a case. The death of a baby was kind of hushed up. It was pretty standard for the baby to be whisked away and the mother encouraged to get pregnant again, as if that could replace the lost child. Nobody wanted to talk to the mother or father about the loss—or they didn't know how. The staff would just come into the room, do what they needed to do, and walk out of the room.

Some years later, I began working in the maternity department. During that time, Terri Zeman started the perinatal loss support group HUGS, which included a seminar for all the staff members. After attending the seminar, I realized that I had never really grieved the loss of my baby, had never gotten the support I needed. That's why it became very important for me to try to help my patients, and that's how I got involved in the effort to create the Garden of Little Angels. I wanted parents to have a healing space where they could go to grieve at the moment of loss, and also a place to return to later—to remember the child that they were never able to watch grow up.

— *Janice Colbert, LPN*
Franklin Square Hospital Center

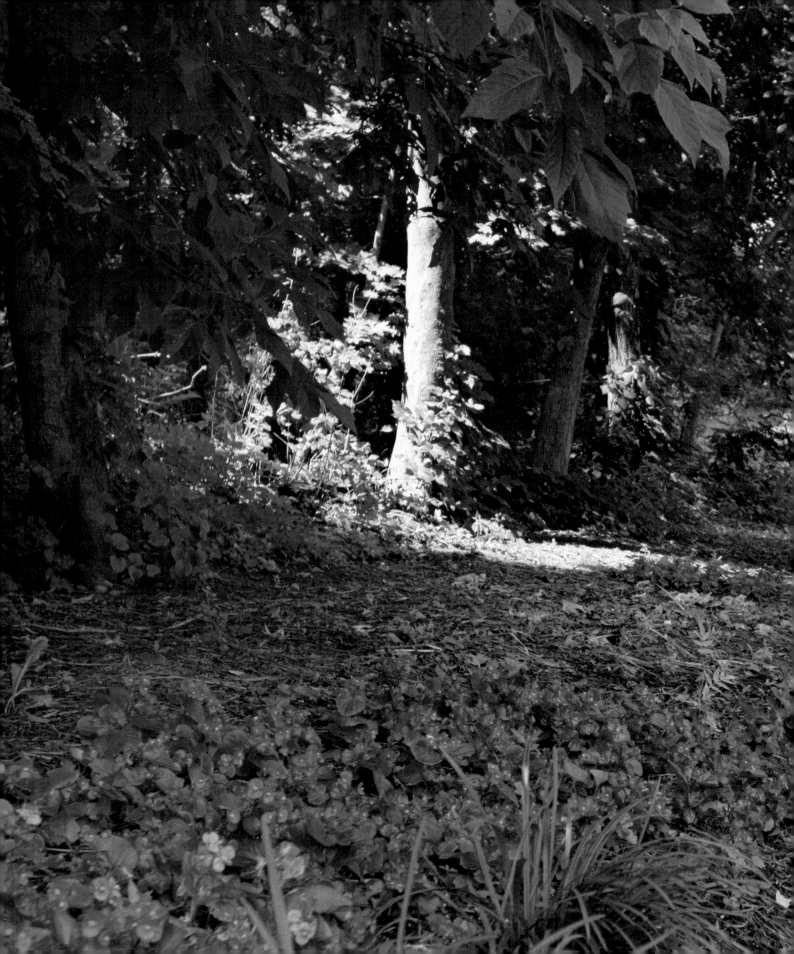

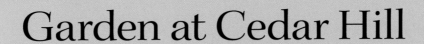 10 Garden at Cedar Hill

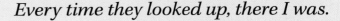

Every time they looked up, there I was.

—Dianne Dale, Firesoul

The breakdown of community, and the subsequent breakdown of institutions, can have an adverse effect on creating a neighborhood garden. Dianne Dale learned this firsthand when she approached her local library on behalf of her garden club.

Dianne lived in Anacostia, a historic African American neighborhood in southeast Washington, D.C. Several generations of her family have called Anacostia home, dating back to the 1890s when Frederick Douglass, former slave and eminent abolitionist, resided in the adjacent community of Uniontown, now the Old Anacostia Historic District. For decades, the neighborhoods thrived. But in her lifetime, Dianne watched as Anacostia slipped from the vibrant, family-focused home of her elders to a shadow of its former self.

Dianne had a dream about the community of her heritage, a dream that she could help restore the respect of the past. One of the ways to achieve that restoration was to create a physical place that her neighbors could point to, a place that they realized in their own time. A garden would tangibly

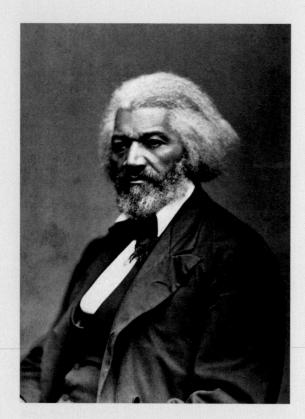

demonstrate, in one small way, a return to the dignity that existed not so long ago. And so it became a question of where to start.

As president of the Anacostia Garden Club, Dianne began by partnering with the local library. The club designed a garden, they raised the money, and then, after several years of hard preparation, they hit a wall. When the community near the library heard that the garden would include a bench, they protested—out of fear of what that bench could attract. Seeing years of hard work disintegrate would cause most people to quit and walk away. Dianne didn't quit. Neither did we at TKF. We told her we would hold onto the grant money. We told her to keep looking.

Four months later, Dianne returned with another idea: build the garden at Cedar Hill, the final home of Frederick Douglass, the community's hero. Cedar Hill is on the National Register of Historic Places, and because it has a federal presence, its grounds are more secure.

Planting a garden at Cedar Hill was no easy task, however. The home, like the neighborhood, was in desperate need of repair. Dianne had to gain access to the land by pushing public officials and community residents to create alliances. She started a nonprofit called Frederick Douglass Gardens Inc., which forged a public/private partnership with the National Park Service (NPS), the entity that oversees Cedar Hill. In 2003, five years after she first approached TKF for grant money for the library project, she finally had permission to plant her garden. One year later, in March 2004, the NPS began a $2.7 million restoration of Douglass' home. Dianne's tenacity to work through the myriad bureaucratic obstacles that blocked her path resulted in a beautiful garden next to a restored Cedar Hill. The wonder of this public/private partnership is that it was the initiative of the community that made it happen. Citizen action right there in Anacostia formed that alliance with the federal government and helped to spur a ripple effect of restoration.

In spite of the success story at Cedar Hill, Dianne is not satisfied. She still has this incredible dream of the community being what it once was. It will take a very long time for Anacostia to come back, but Dianne was willing to take a first step. How many people, knowing how long the road may be, are willing to take that first step? When you think of all the dangerous parks in this country, all the degradation that's just down the block, it's amazing to realize that through your own initiative, you can do something. Dianne Dale is living proof.

—*T.S.*

Dianne Dale

President, Frederick Douglass Gardens Inc. and Community Historian

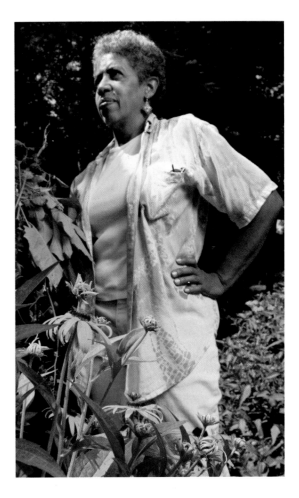

Flowers show you care. That's what Mrs. Murray, who founded the Anacostia Garden Club eighteen years ago, always says. I agree. And somebody has to care about our neighborhood, because it has been on a steady decline for about sixty years.

Our neighborhood is Anacostia, a community in the southeast sector of Washington, D.C. This is the neighborhood where Frederick Douglass, the great African American orator and writer, lived more than a century ago. Today, his home is designated a national historic site. During his lifetime, there were two neighboring communities in Anacostia—one white, one black. Frederick Douglass lived in the white community, and he was the first black to purchase property there. But Frederick Douglass was still involved in the black community. His three sons lived in black Anacostia. However, the community that was thriving when he lived here, and fifty years into the next century, has degenerated into a slum.

For nearly twenty-five years, I've been involved in various ways to try to restore the dignity and respect this community once had. One of those ways was through the garden club. When I was growing up here, this was a neighborhood of mostly single-family homes, and most of the owners planted gardens. They took pride in what they had, and their gardens demonstrated that pride. So while I was president of the garden club, we committed to planting a garden on the grounds of Cedar Hill, the Frederick Douglass home. We wanted to demonstrate, by creating a beautiful space, that some people still care and that our historic neighborhood is worth caring about.

I wasn't always a community activist. When I was growing up in Anacostia, it was a good place to live. But things began to go downhill in the 1950s. I moved to Florida for a job, and every time I returned to visit my family, I could see the decline. I'd come home and think, "It can't get any worse than

Sun setting over my shoulder
Ground frozen
Toes frozen
Silence amidst the traffic
Stillness within the storm
Thank you for this moment
Our journey just begins.

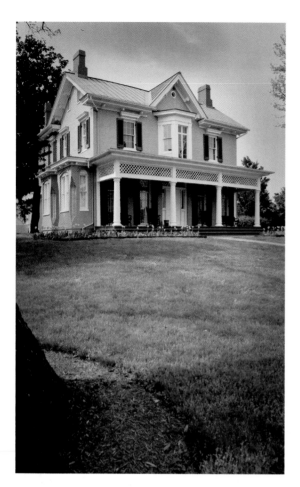

this." And every time I came back, it was worse. When my father died in 1984, I came home for his funeral with the intention of returning to Florida. But I looked around me and thought, "My father worked too hard for it to come to this. His parents and grandparents and all the folks who put so much effort into creating a good place to live—it's not right, it's just not right." So I never went back to Florida.

Anacostia has a rich history, including the Revolutionary War and the Civil War; in 1954, this black community was one of the parties to Brown v. Board of Education. Frederick Douglass was our local hero. His home sits high on a hill with a spectacular view of the U.S. Capitol, the Washington Monument, the National Cathedral, and the grand sweep of the capital's wide avenues. He used the grounds of his home to contemplate the issues of the day and to find respite and peace. Before his home became part of the National Park Service in 1970, the community took care of the house and gardens. We had raffles to buy supplies and paid kids in the neighborhood to paint his house. Cub Scouts helped take care of the grounds.

But Anacostia's history didn't start with Frederick Douglass. When Douglass moved here in 1877, he moved next to a thriving African American community of about 1,500 people, established a decade before by the Freedmen's Bureau. Education was highly valued: one of the first things the new community did was build a school. Black Anacostia was a village where everyone knew everyone else, and parents watched out for all neighborhood children. They did what was best for the children and for the community ethic. My great-grandparents came here in the 1890s, while Frederick Douglass

I live near here. The city as a vibrant place is important to me. Always, every day, I hear and see more and more ugliness . . . This spot reminds me that we can and must continue to struggle for the good, the beautiful, and the peaceful in life. Thank you!

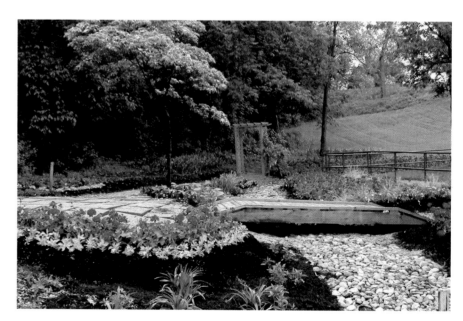

was still living in the adjacent white community, and my family instilled in me the kind of community pride we all felt at being a special part of the city's history and of black history. But then things started to decline. Today there are two, maybe three, generations living in Anacostia who know nothing of this history.

The change began in the 1940s, when black servicemen were coming back from World War II. Housing for them and their families was difficult to find. The Roosevelt administration had built housing in Appalachia for distressed populations. Following that model, several war housing projects were built in our community, with the government either condemning the land or taking it by eminent domain. Bolling Air Force Base was built on some of our land, and a four-lane parkway was added, running directly from the south entrance of the Capitol to the air force base. The parkway made it easy for dignitaries to get back and forth, but it split our community right down the middle. When highways were being built during the Eisenhower years, an interstate sliced up our community even more.

In the 1950s, the zoning was changed to allow only multi-family dwellings to be built, and that sounded a death-knell for our greenspace. They scraped it all away and built thousands of "garden apartments," which is a misnomer: the renters who moved into them had little interest in planting gardens. All this activity chopped up Anacostia and destroyed a way of life. Then came desegregation in 1954, which destroyed our excellent schools and caused large numbers of people, both white and black, to migrate to the suburbs. In 1987, the District of Columbia built a subway line through the area, and Metro construction destroyed the last remaining part of the community that was intact, including eleven lovely old homes.

The community that my father was born in and built was gone, and the generations who have lived here since never knew that way of life. They have no sense of the rich history, and I believe a sense of history is what helps develop our self-image. My generation is the last to know the story of what the community once was. As I worked in various capacities—in the schools, on the Advisory Neighborhood Commission, in the garden club—I began to feel more and more strongly that the story needed to be told, so I put the history of the area together in a book called *Mark the Place: Voices of an Invisible Community.*

Then something happened in 1997 that blasted me into action. There is a sixty-acre section of our community called Poplar Point, which sits right on the Anacostia River. It was once a part of the black community, privately owned by residents, and it was taken when the federal government reclaimed

No signs, no fences, no restrictions. Just a lovely place to sit.

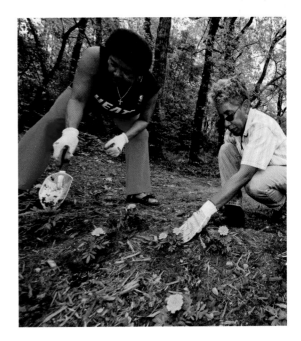

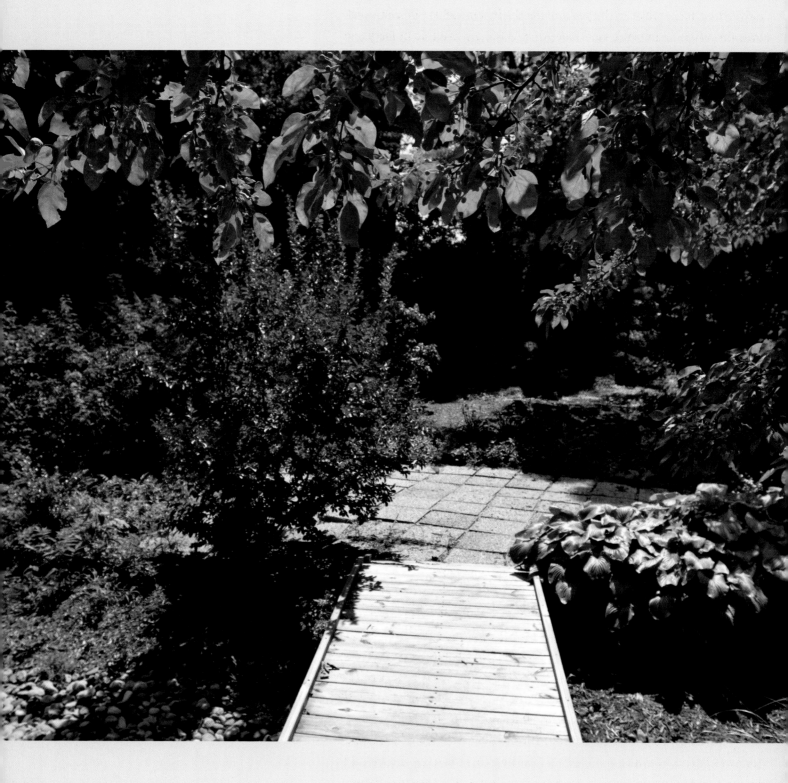

the waterfront. The government dredged the river and filled it in to create a riverfront park similar to the parks along the Potomac River in southwest Washington. It became the site of the Architect of the Capitol's nursery and the D.C. Tree Nursery. In 1997, the City announced plans to pave over that sixty acres and make it a Metro parking lot for commuters. Asphalt! Can you imagine? That's when I said, "No. We can't let this happen." Then someone from the community who was also outraged came to our garden club and suggested that we create a garden on that land, as well as a memorial to Frederick Douglass. And that's how it all started.

We had a beautiful vision for those sixty acres at Poplar Point. We wanted to create something like the National Arboretum, with trees, shrubs, flowers, and walkways. But we quickly realized that this was more of a pipe dream than a plan. However, thinking and talking about this resulted in my getting in touch with the TKF Foundation.

TKF encouraged, and ultimately funded, the creation of a smaller garden for the community. We went first to the local library, but that did not work out: there was concern that a bench would attract "unsavory" types. We had no intention of planting a contemplative garden and not putting in a TKF bench where people could come and sit, so we moved on—looking next at the grounds surrounding Frederick Douglass' Cedar Hill home. At this time, many of the national parks were suffering from lack of funding, and the Frederick Douglass National Historic Site had fallen into such disrepair that it was listed as one of the Ten Most Endangered National Parks. "Why not here?" we thought. "It needs as much help as anything in the community."

So I went to the superintendent of National Capital Parks East and said, "I have the money to put in a garden. Do you want one?" He did—but the house needed so many repairs that he was afraid a garden would spread the already-thin resources even thinner. We negotiated and presented a plan for the garden and finally signed a contract. In 2000, we incorporated a new organization—Frederick Douglass Gardens Inc.—which of course, had no money, so I continued to handle the negotiations and paperwork. When we started creating the garden during the fall of 2002, a lot of the work was done by garden club volunteers. We came back in the spring to plant the annuals. Shortly after that, once the site manager saw how the lovely gardens added to the visitors' experience of the home, she put the garden in the annual budget. That budgeted money pays for the annuals, but I and some other club members still tend the garden. We were very careful when we chose the trees, shrubs, and plants, to put things in that Mother Nature could take care of without our

As people hurry about rushing to work on a Monday morning, pushing and shoving their way through the Metro doors with no excuses given for their rude behavior, this garden near everything but yet so far away brings a sense of peace to my day.

Do not be impatient. Sit quietly and perhaps a butterfly will light upon you.

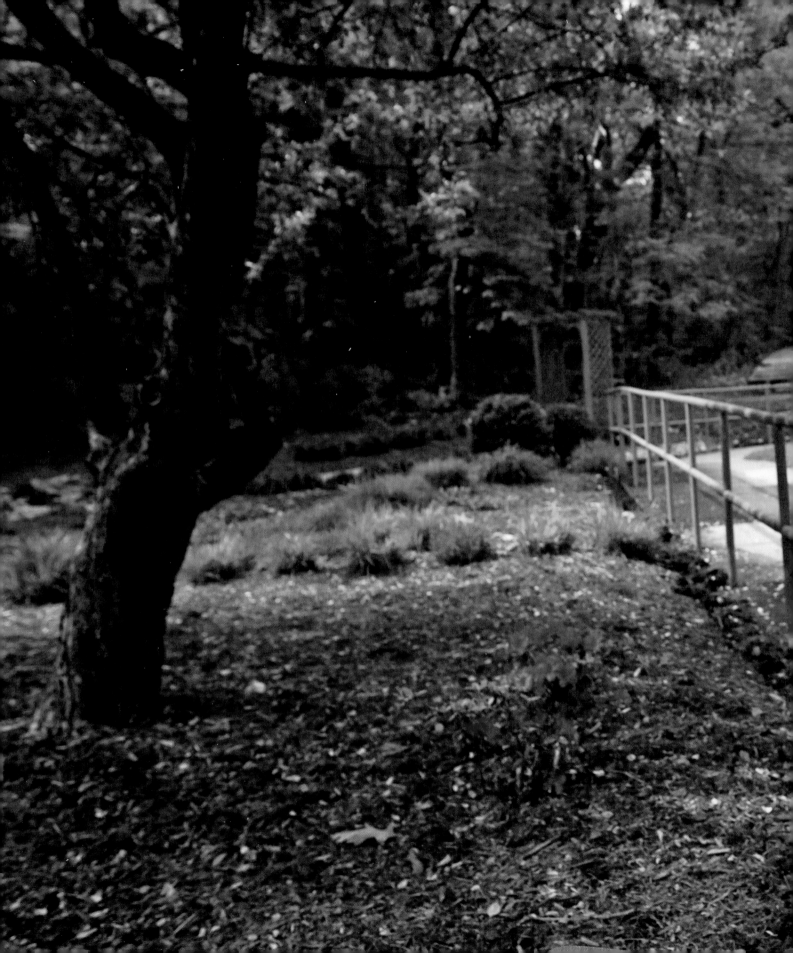

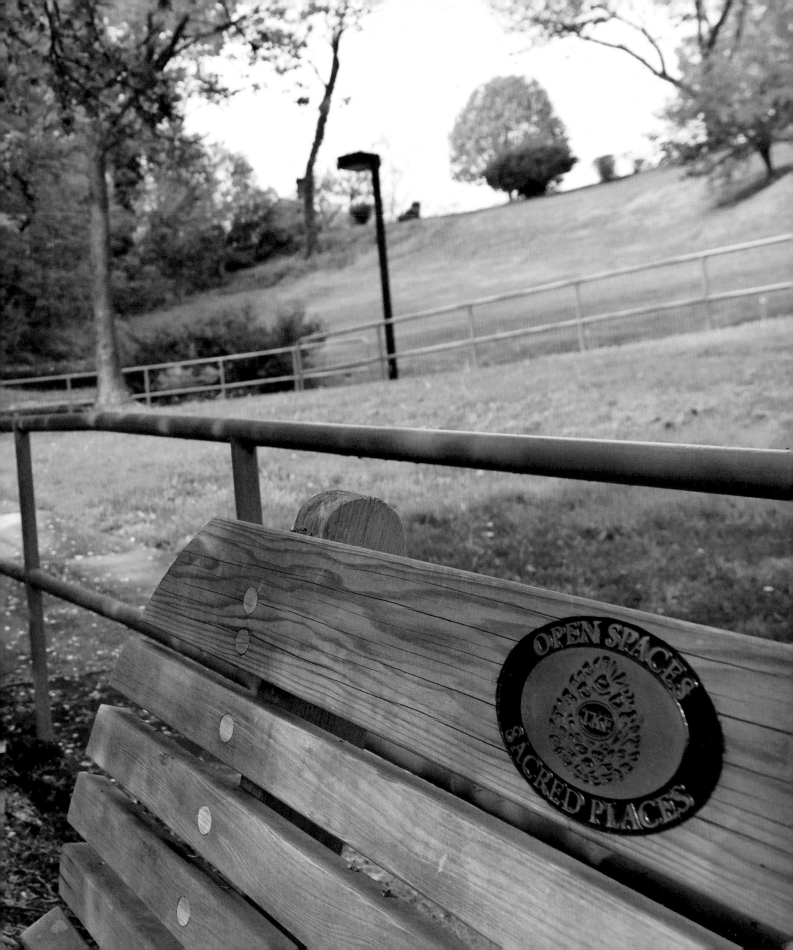

Although the sounds of sirens, helicopter blades, and honking horns are heard, the early morning dew, crickets' legs rubbing, and birds singing their song somehow drown out those everyday noises and make me feel that my day has just begun with new wonders to see and new dreams to search for.

Within everyone's soul is the voice of God seeking permission to speak.

help, including a lot of native plants that are drought-resistant. But it is still a job to take care of it.

One of the things the National Park Service did when they took over the site in 1970 was put a fence around the Frederick Douglass house, which immediately took away community access to the land and the feeling of community ownership. I think the gardens open up the space again and say, "Come in. You're welcome." We involve people from the community in caring for the garden too, so they can feel some ownership. The Earth Conservation Corps (ECC) brought a crew, which included some young folks from our neighborhood, to help install the garden. The ECC is essentially an environmental job corps that trains kids in distressed circumstances to be environmental stewards and encourages them to earn a GED if they don't have a high school diploma.

We've gotten schools involved, too—elementary, middle, and high schools. We had intended to have school children help with the garden installation, but that was the autumn that the sniper was terrorizing the Washington metropolitan area, and we couldn't take the chance. Every spring, the school children come and help plant the annuals, and we say to them, "This is your garden. These are your flowers. You've done this." And if we have a child who is really interested, we give him or her a plant to take home. Sometimes the children come with their parents. That's wonderful, because it reaches into another layer of the community. We invite visitors to actually take part in the garden, by inviting them to pull a weed if they see one. I hope—I think—the gardens are drawing people from the neighborhood to the historic site, which is a sort of backdoor way of connecting them to their own history. And the garden is a very visible, very tangible way of showing respect for that history, part of our effort to reestablish the reputation of the community.

We stand at a dangerous moment, a moment when we could lose so much because Anacostia has been "discovered." It's the last frontier of Washington, D.C., if you will—the views are magnificent, the land is cheaper, and it's convenient to every place from Richmond to New York City. Because most of the current residents of Anacostia have seen nothing but decline in their lifetimes, they are much more apt to accept anything new that's offered to the community—a soccer stadium on the waterfront or even a parking lot—just so long as the run-down stuff is gone. They're desperate, and that's when decisions are made that are not in the best long-term interest of the community. At Poplar Point, for example, developers are fighting to pass zoning that would allow eight-story buildings. They might be nice for the few people who live in them, but the buildings would completely block the wonderful views that right now belong to the whole community. These views are so much a part of the community that people take them for granted, but if the views disappear, people are not going to feel as good and probably won't even know why. These changes can be so gradual that you don't recognize what's happening until you've lost what you had and can never get it back. And as far as I'm concerned, that's stealing from the community.

I've learned two really important things from my experience with the gardens over the last ten years. First, I've gained the confidence needed to get things done in a bureaucracy. Second, I've learned to be both persistent and patient. It may take a long time, but if you keep showing up, they have to deal with you. The Park Service had to understand that I was serious about creating that garden at Poplar Point, and the only way I could prove that was to keep showing up. Every time they looked up, there I was.

Much to my disappointment, the city has chosen a company to redevelop Poplar Point. But it is still important to me that its historic significance is not obliterated. And because we prevailed in our effort to put the garden in at Cedar Hill, I am determined to establish a treasured greenspace at Poplar Point. There *will* be a garden there because in 2005, the National Capital Memorial Advisory Commission approved a request from Frederick Douglass Gardens Inc. for five acres at Poplar Point. What else will happen is uncertain at this point, but on those five acres, there will be a memorial park and a garden that celebrates the community, the one that Frederick Douglass lived in, the one that generations of my family helped build, the one where I grew up.

Recently, when I was working over at the Cedar Hill gardens, I sat down on the TKF bench and leafed through the journal to see what people had written. There was an entry from a graduate of nearby Howard University. She was pondering the black condition, and she wrote, "What in the world would Frederick Douglass be thinking if he were to come back today and see what his neighborhood has become?" I've wondered that myself over the years, especially twenty-three years ago when I came back for my father's funeral. But if Frederick Douglass were to come back right now and sit here in this beautiful garden beside his restored home, he might think, "There's hope." I know I do.

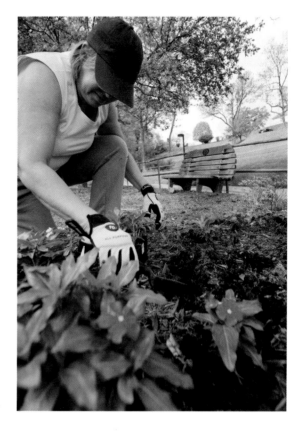

I am going to believe in myself today and make something happen. It's time.

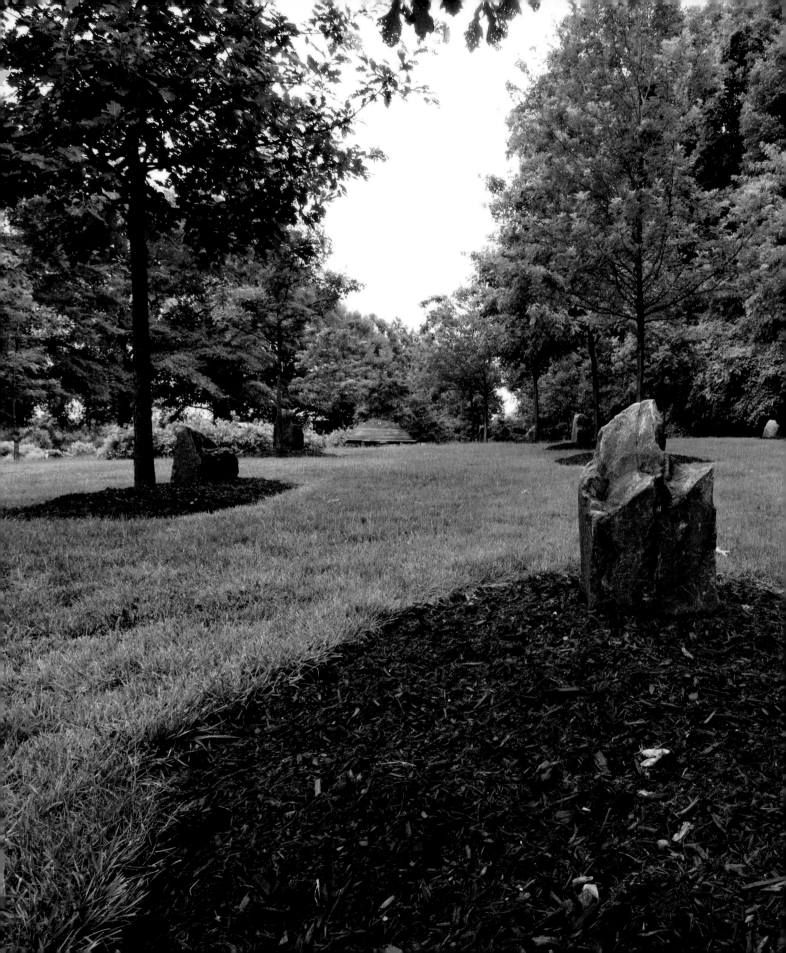

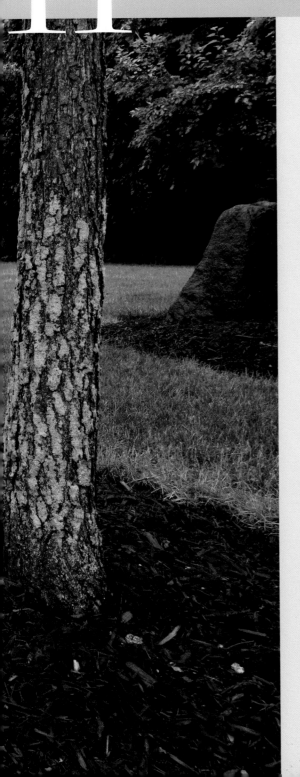

11 Joseph Beuys Tree Partnership: *7000 Oaks*

We Americans are pragmatic. We forget the importance of poetry in our lives, of quiet time.

— Renee van der Stelt, Firesoul

Sometimes, a global vision can inspire a local intervention. In this case, inspiration came from a brilliant outdoor sculpture project by German artist Joseph Beuys, one of the most important artists of the twentieth century. The original project, called *7000 Oaks,* began at Documenta 7, an international art exhibition in Kassel, Germany. Between 1982 and 1987, Beuys involved the entire Kassel community in the planning and planting of seven thousand oak trees, paired with seven thousand basalt stones from a nearby volcanic quarry. The ever-changing symbiotic relationship of the stones and trees transformed the community's attitudes toward the environment and brought reforestation to the area. The citywide project also gave Beuys the opportunity to address his social concerns: to improve the ecosystem, develop positive economic and political voices in an urban setting, and improve life for all in the city. Most important, he invited others to expand on his work, in other sites throughout the world. Beyond the living legacy of those thousands of new trees, Beuys opened up the definition of *creativity* and encouraged others to see how they could change the world through their own actions.

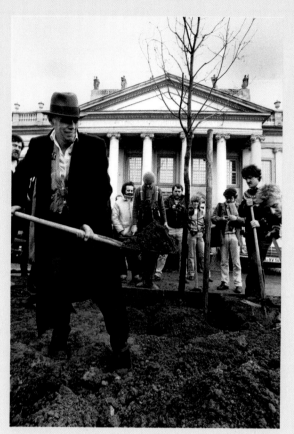

Renee van der Stelt, museum educator at the University of Maryland Baltimore County (UMBC), felt impelled to take up that call and bring Beuys' inspiration to her campus and her adopted city of Baltimore. The artist and teacher built bridges within the university and opened up a line of communication with the surrounding city. She forged a partnership with local agencies, like the city Department of Recreation and Parks, and she brought hundreds of students from both the university and the inner city together to create what Beuys called "a social sculpture." The magnitude of the project seemed impossible at first. The first phase of the Joseph Beuys Tree Partnership would see the planting of 212 indigenous trees in three city parks, and thirty oak trees and thirty stones placed at UMBC. But by using the combined power of both communities, Renee proved the truth of Beuys' belief that every human being is an artist and that when empowered, every individual can accomplish amazing feats. Baltimore now joins the list of urban centers worldwide to embrace Beuys' ideas.

The writings recorded in journals located within the UMBC site serve as compelling testimony to the positive power of nature to inspire new generations of users of sacred spaces. The writings serve to hearten those who maintain the space and to communicate the continued value and importance of keeping greenspaces open. The Joseph Beuys Tree Partnership ensures that the community not only has room to breathe, but also has a place to connect to nature and to cultivate individual creativity.

—T.S.

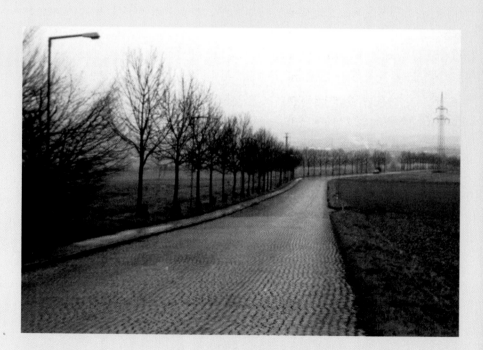

Renee van der Stelt

Museum Educator and Registrar, Center for Art
and Individual Culture at UMBC

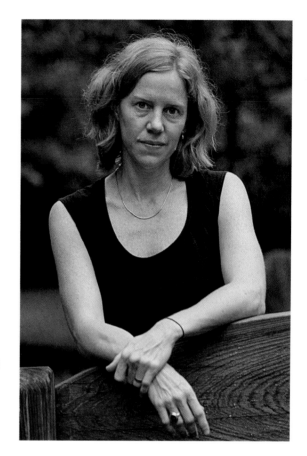

I was exposed to the work and philosophy of Joseph Beuys when I worked at the Walker Art Center in Minneapolis. I was attracted immediately. Beuys was a political activist as well as an artist, and his art—especially his *7000 Oaks* project—engaged both my sense of social justice and my deep desire to care for the environment. The really wonderful thing about *7000 Oaks* is that Beuys left it open-ended, so that anyone anywhere could take it up at anytime and plant trees with the goal of regenerating urban landscapes.

In one sense, my motivation to take on this project was quite personal: I wanted more city greenspace so that I could bike more. I had biked all the time in Minneapolis, and when I moved to Baltimore in 1999, I was distressed that there were so few places for me to do what I loved. At that time, the City was just beginning to talk about a greenway, and the parks were in dire straits because of budget cuts. Baltimore felt like a city of concrete compared to Minneapolis. I missed the green open spaces desperately. It got me thinking about how to make a city a more livable space. One way, of course, is by planting trees—and that took me right back to Beuys' *7000 Oaks* project.

But beyond just planting trees, Beuys had an intense sense of social justice—the same sense of social justice that was instilled in me during my childhood. I grew up in a Calvinist Dutch immigrant home, with a father who is a minister and a philosopher, and I was raised with the idea "Do unto others as you would have them do unto you." Obviously, that includes major rules like "Do not kill." But for me, it also means that if you want to create a beautiful space, that space should be created for and open to everyone, no matter what his or her economic standing may be.

There is no ego amidst these trees.
There is no bravado.
There is no "only one way."
Trees don't know war.

I knew that other cities and art centers had completed tree projects modeled on *7000 Oaks*. There were projects in New York City, Minneapolis, and Omaha in the United States, as well as in Oslo, Norway, and Sydney, Australia. The more I thought about doing a tree project in Baltimore, the more exciting the idea became. I felt that it would bring together so many parts of my life.

First, the project has a strong environmental component. Growing up in Iowa, I was surrounded by farmers. They talked about land use, about "corn or soybeans, soybeans or corn"; they talked about how we'd lost 40 percent of the rich topsoil that used to grow bluegrass and had supported humans for centuries. All my life I've been aware of our need and responsibility to care for the earth, and Beuys' work helped me to see how I could use art to do that.

As an artist, these are the big questions for me: What are artists doing to make their work relevant? How are they applying their knowledge to what's going on around us? Beuys made *7000 Oaks* relevant by involving the citizens of Kassel. The city had been decimated by bombing in World War II. By having the community residents plant the trees, Beuys gave the people an opportunity to be part of the revitalization of their city. Through their participation, they became aware of the need for each individual to take action on behalf of the earth. Certainly, that need is becoming more urgent as we learn more about global warming, but Beuys was very forward-thinking: he was using his art to involve citizens in this important work decades ago. The thought of involving the people of Baltimore in planting trees intrigued me.

Age is inevitable; growth is optional.

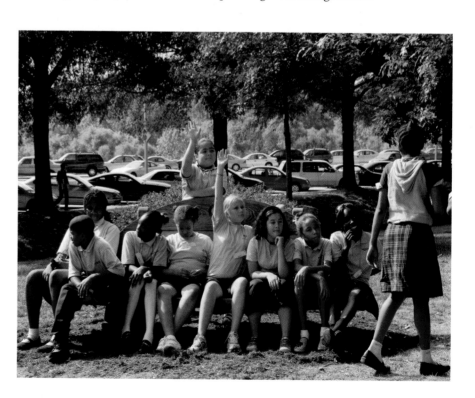

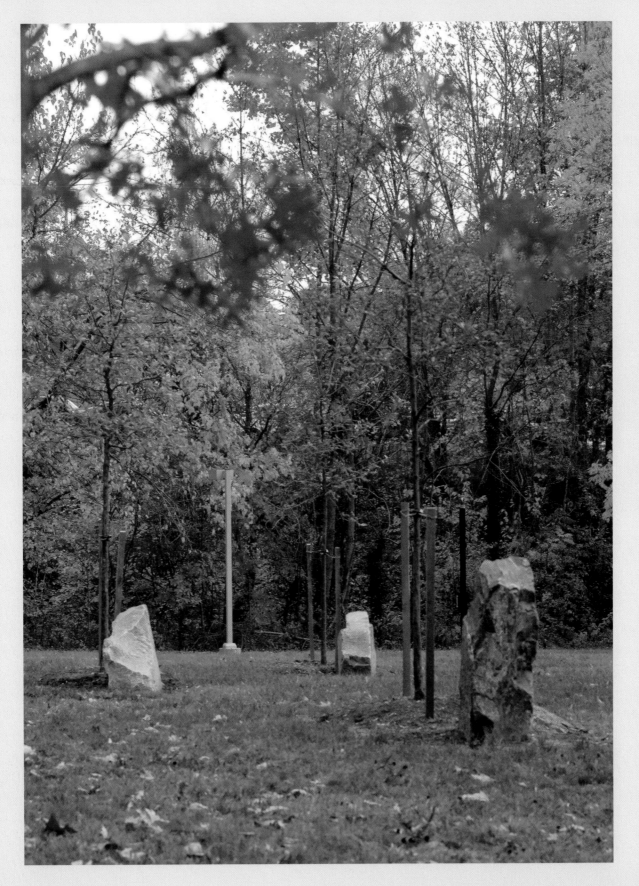

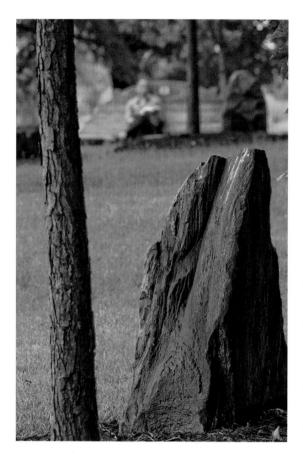

What a wonderful idea. At first, I didn't like the association of a stone with a tree. But now I understand the symbolism behind it. Now every time I see the garden, it will no longer look like a graveyard, but it will remind me to grow.

Another benefit of this involvement—of what Beuys calls "social sculpture"—is the possibility of changing the way people view themselves. He said, "The true capital of the world is the human ability for creativity, freedom, and self-determination in all their working places." I love that quote because we live in a capitalist, money-driven society, and Beuys takes the idea of *capital* and turns it on its head. He is saying that what really matters is not monetary, but the human heart and human action, and I agree. I was very excited to see what would happen to people if they came to view the act of planting a tree as a creative act and to view themselves as artists. Most people don't take ownership of their creativity. They think, "I can't draw; therefore, I'm not an artist, and I'm not creative." But Beuys tried to get people to broaden the definition of *creative,* which, of course, would give them a much broader range of options for participating creatively in the world around them.

Finally, I wanted to create quiet space in the city—a place where people could be reflective and feel more connected to nature. We Americans are pragmatic. We forget the importance of poetry in our lives, of quiet time, of peace-filled alone time when things shift and come together because we have taken the time to reflect on our lives. I love silence. I grew up in a small rural town, and although I didn't know it, I was mostly surrounded by silence. Out of that silence, I developed a relationship with nature. When I moved to the city, I felt an incredible sadness at the loss not only of the silence, but of the "conversations" I'd had with nature, such as listening to the wind in the trees. For instance, the wind sounds louder in October than in September, because the leaves are drier. I wanted to create a space where people could have the experience of listening to nature.

So with all these thoughts motivating me, I began to search for funding and discovered TKF. Not only was TKF interested in my project, they urged me to expand my modest proposal. The result is Baltimore's Joseph Beuys Tree Partnership, which involved twenty-one partner organizations and more than five hundred people planting a total of 242 trees, in three parks and on UMBC's campus.

We chose the park sites carefully. The urban community's involvement was vital for the success of the project. We wanted to encourage people to have hope for their parks and immediate environment and to promote the concept of healing and creative action through the planting of trees. In doing this project, the Fine Arts Gallery (now the Center for Art and Visual Culture) at UMBC tried to step beyond the traditional gallery walls to show that the arts are not for the privileged elite, but rather that they are woven into the daily fabric of life.

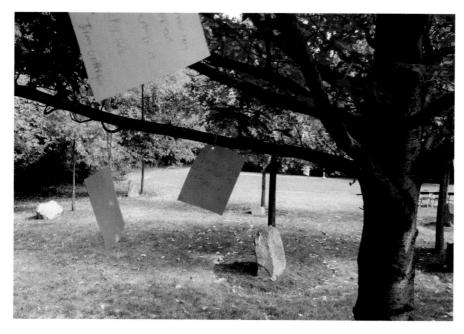

*The purpose of life is simple.
It is to discover the gift you were
endowed with, develop it, then return it.*

We especially wanted to attract children, so that they could take ownership in improving their own neighborhoods and so that we could use the project to provide education and plant the seeds to grow future conservationists.
We chose three parks that had schools in close proximity and were located in
economically disadvantaged neighborhoods, where planting trees had the potential to vastly improve the daily environment of the residents. The teachers
helped by bringing students to the parks to plant trees—a hundred trees each
at two of the parks and twelve trees at a third, with granite stones placed next
to an oak tree in each park. It was wonderful to watch. A lot of the children

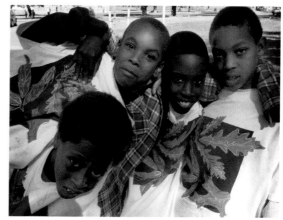

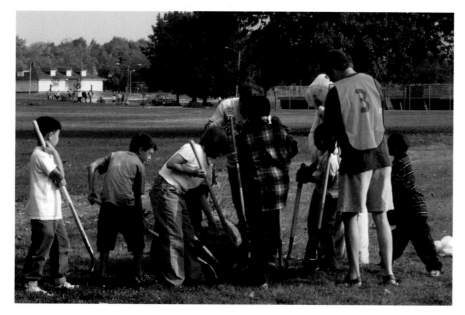

*A love for things beautiful brought me here
today. Love that can be traced back to the
beginning of time when there was just man
and nature.*

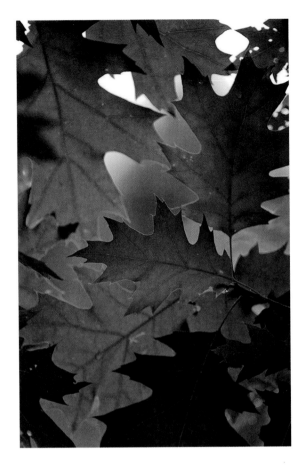

had never had their hands in the dirt before, which amazed me. Every time they encountered a worm, they broke out into uncontrollable giggles. At each site, we held a special ceremony that celebrated the revitalized landscape.

We sent some UMBC art students to work with the teachers to help the children create visual art projects based on the ideas of Joseph Beuys and greening. Over the next six to eight weeks, the children created artwork. Meanwhile on the UMBC campus, university students helped to plant thirty oak trees and place thirty granite stones next to them, creating the first public sculpture project at the university. We then brought the children's artwork to UMBC for an exhibition. The children and their parents came to see the artwork and also to see the newly created Beuys Sculpture Park at UMBC. This event was an extremely important part of the project. Most of the children were city kids who had never been to a university. We showed them a way that their education could continue. This piece tied in with my own desire for educational social justice, because inner city children often don't get the highest quality education.

The Beuys Sculpture Park at UMBC encompasses all of Beuys' elements and most clearly shows the symbiotic relationship of the trees and stones. For *7000 Oaks,* Beuys selected the oak tree and the basalt stone—two elements with inherent beauty—and set them next to each other in a symbolic action. Initially, when the tree and stone are planted side by side, the stone dwarfs the tree. But over time, the tree dwarfs the stone, and the stone is diminished, letting its minerals seep into the ground and feed the roots of the tree. The tree and stone therefore become symbols for the human activity of creative regeneration and for the connectedness of life in the environment. Beuys focused on

The last page of the book, to be treasured always. A peaceful place for those who wish to think. A friendly place for those who wish to chill. The rock garden is created with every person's intention in mind.

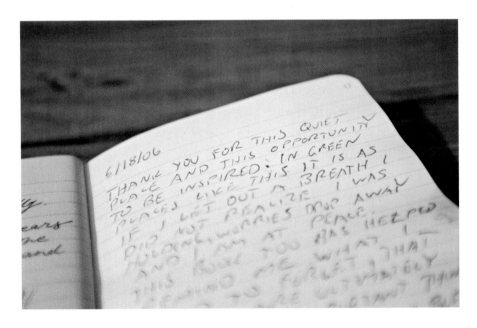

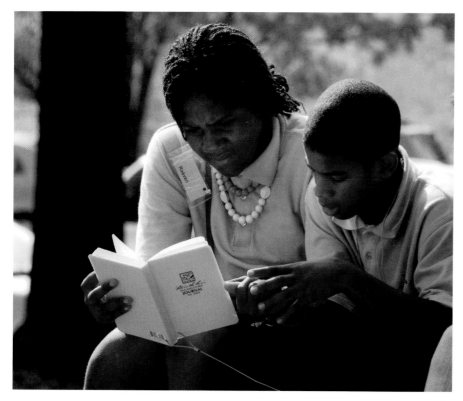

Don't you think it's weird how a little plastic yellow book can connect a whole bunch of people together? . . . I hope you are all doing alright. I'll be back to check up on everyone soon.

the urban setting because he understood that it is in the city that life is often most alienated from the natural environment.

We planted all oaks at the UMBC site because that is the tree that Beuys chose. Oaks are slow-growing, they have a very solid heartwood, and their roots go as deep as their branches grow wide. We chose thirty stones from a nearby granite quarry. They vary in shape and are quite lovely. In the seven years since the sculpture was planted, the trees have doubled in size, demonstrating the ever-changing nature of our surroundings and the need for us to be aware of the continual care our environment needs.

We know that our spirits also need care, so in the center of the trees is a TKF bench with a journal. The journal entries tell us that the space is being used in the way we had hoped. Students write in the journal, but there are also a number of entries from people who visit from the community. The writings come from evening hours as well as daytime—we know that from people describing what they see as they sit and look up at the sky. Many of the entries express gratitude for a place to sit and ponder. Some express happiness, others loneliness. We've filled many journals and have sent copies of the entries to the president of the university, who loves reading them and has been very supportive of the site. I think the journal entries have encouraged him to

This book, too, has helped remind me what I tend to forget, that people are ultimately the most important things in our lives. How blessed I am to be surrounded and supported by so many good people. Life is good. I am at peace.

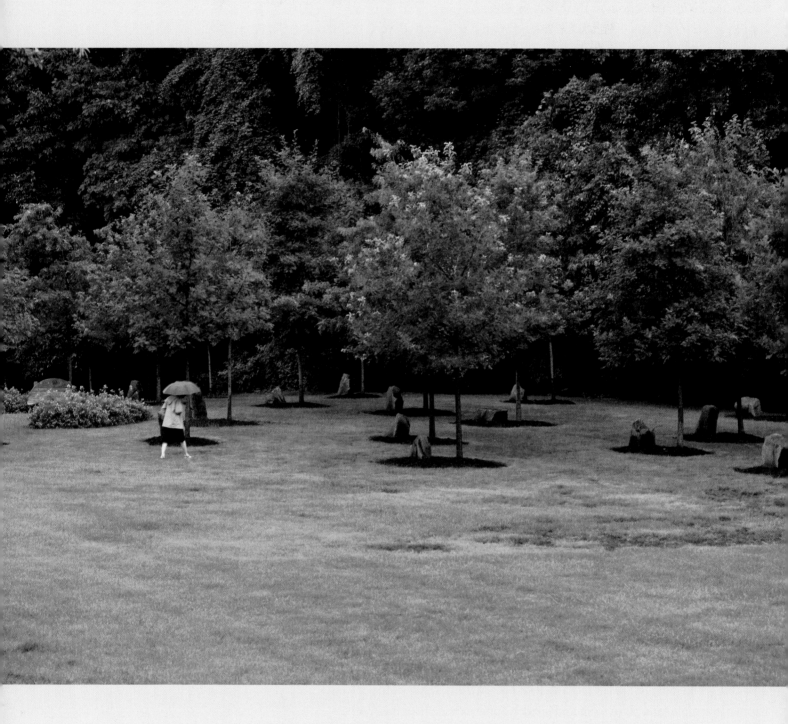

think about creating more greenspaces on campus and building a stronger campus community—by making him aware of the thoughts and feelings of the student body that he would not otherwise know.

It has been such fun to watch the trees grow and change from year to year. Maintenance, of course, is part of every living sculpture, so TKF counseled us to incorporate tree maintenance into our budget. Because of this, we've had good results with the trees and have needed to replace very few. The spirit of cooperation from the Department of Recreation and Parks has been generous and strong. The project would not have been successful without the support of the city organizations and the hundreds of people who helped plant the trees.

In the years since I moved to Baltimore, the City has made a huge commitment to greening and tree planting. For instance, in 2006, it launched a program to double its tree canopy. I continue to be inspired by organizations that are interested in building new partnerships to keep on greening the city and strengthening the many communities within it. To bring my own story full circle, the beautiful fourteen-mile biking and hiking Gwynn Falls Trail has opened, and I can now bike three-fourths of my way to work on it.

When Joseph Beuys started his *7000 Oaks* project, he printed postcards to build support for it. The first card had an image of an oak tree and said, "Let your ideas take root." We did that. The second had an image of a stone and said, "Put your stone in motion." I believe he understood that people are inherently static and need to be invited to action. We did that. The third one had a coin on it and said, "Every tree has a price." Beuys was talking about the monetary price of greening urban areas, but also about the price—the challenge—of organizing the many people it takes to keep a place green and to stop it from being cemented over. We did that—and I'd like to think that the Joseph Beuys Tree Partnership helped to generate some of the community interest and impetus for the exciting things that are taking place today to make Baltimore greener and more livable.

At the outset of this project, my friend—who is the founder of the Center for Social Sculpture and who was in charge of the *7000 Oaks* project in northern Minnesota—told me that planting a tree is a spiritual act. Today, I stand convinced of this.

Ryan got down on one knee and proposed to the love of his life, Lisa. She accepted, and now they officially begin their lives together.

I'm just glad the book exists and that you found it to write in, because when I'm feeling really emotional, it feels good to know others are out there feeling the same thing.

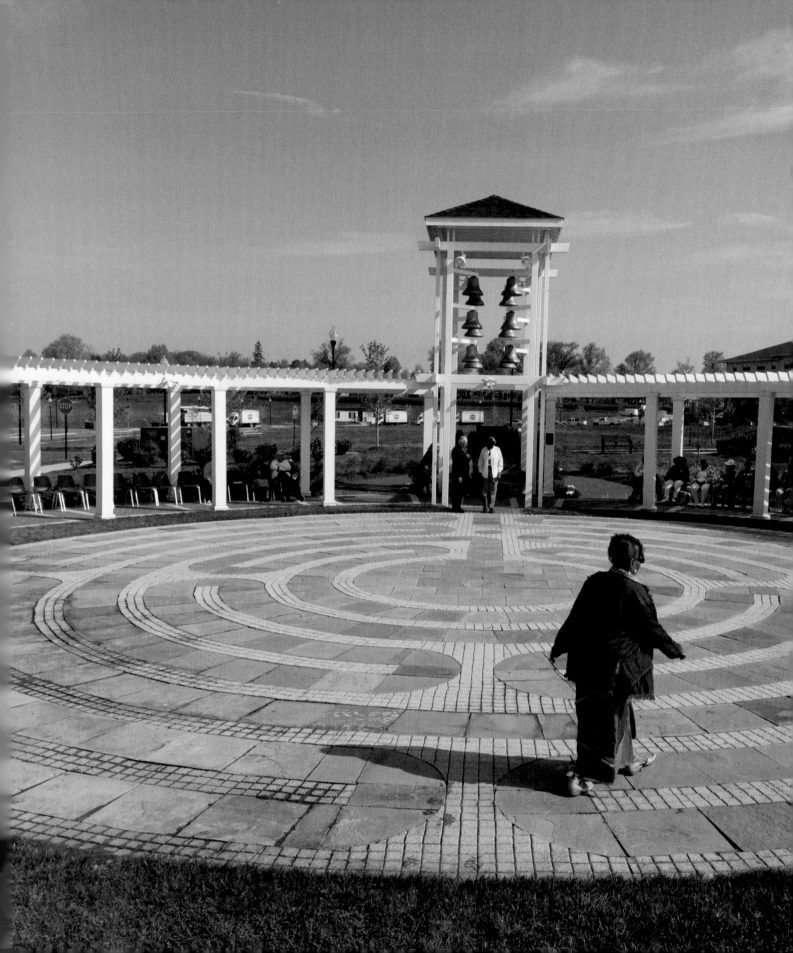

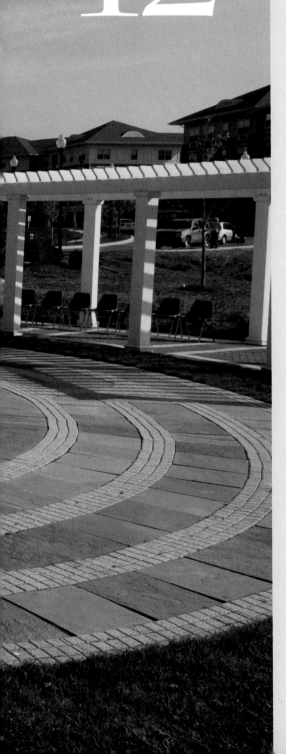

12 ThanksGiving Place

He said to me, 'I've been watching you, Jack, and you're off to a good start. But don't be a flash in the pan.'

—Jack Sharp, Firesoul

In 1999, Reverend Jack Sharp achieved the unbelievable. A Presbyterian pastor, Jack, along with an interfaith team of community leaders, went up against some of the biggest developers in the country to bid on thirty-three acres in Baltimore. Once the hub of community activity, where thousands cheered the Orioles and the Colts at Memorial Stadium, the site needed a fresh life, now that the sports teams were in new stadiums downtown. Jack and his colleagues had a vision for a neighborhood, including affordable senior housing and a YMCA for youth services. He believed that bringing generations together creates something very special, and he wanted to again make this area a place of kinship and vibrancy. Against the odds, Jack Sharp and his team won. Today, Stadium Place is a reality.

But Jack wanted to do more than create facilities to serve multiple generations. He also wanted to create a space that could serve all spiritual paths. He has an uncanny ability to meet people where they are: he is devoted to his faith, yet open to all. So when community member Susan MacFarlane suggested creating an open space around the idea of thanksgiving, Jack embraced it. Susan had been inspired by Thanks-Giving Square in Dallas, Texas, and by the Angel of Thanksgiving in Belfast,

171

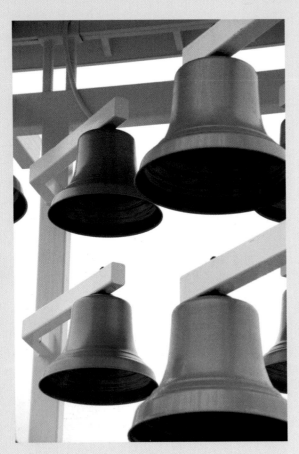

Ireland. She believes that gratitude and the spirit of thanksgiving have the power to heal. Thanksgiving is universal; it's in every religion. Having gratitude represents the human spirit at its finest moment.

ThanksGiving Place is now the spiritual center of the community. The design includes a portal that transports visitors from the city outside to the sacred labyrinth inside. The blue flagstone labyrinth is the heart of ThanksGiving Place. A carillon, a memorial to a beloved city councilman, stands at the entrance to the labyrinth. The carillon, which is electronic, can be used to play a wide variety of music, from many cultures and faiths. It seems a fitting metaphor: different sounds working together for a more beautiful whole. The carillon creates a universal calling for the community to come together.

In our culture and time, many of us are turned inward. But the idea of gratitude implies thinking about somebody else, and therefore, thinking about the community. By bringing people together around a collective experience, around the idea of gratitude, ThanksGiving Place creates a unifying force. Anyone and everyone may participate, and every individual is a part of the whole.

—*T.S.*

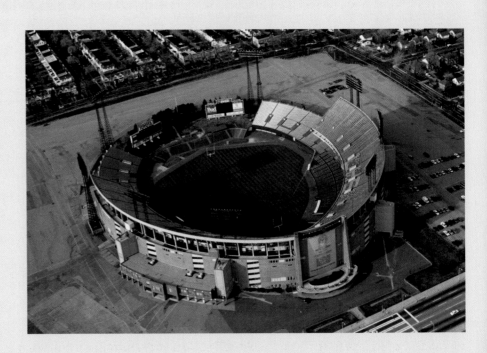

Jack Sharp

President, ThanksGiving Place

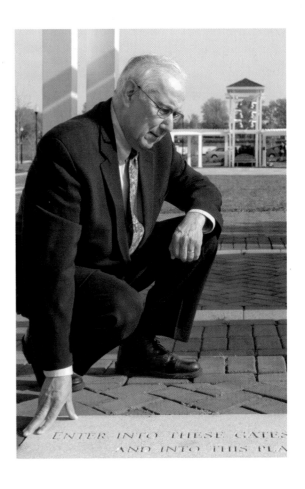

It was decades ago, but I'll never forget what someone said to me when I was a young minister in Newark, New Jersey. On the day I was admitted to the presbytery, a day when most people were congratulating me, a Portuguese pastor who was very committed to community projects came up to me and said, "I've been watching you, Jack, and you're off to a good start. But don't be a flash in the pan. If you start something, finish it. Don't quit when the going gets hard."

His words made a deep impression on me, and I've thought of him during the years that I've been involved in the interfaith effort to create affordable housing for low-income seniors. It has been a long road, and it has been tough at times. But we all held to our vision, and here we are. Over the years, the number of congregational and community supporters has grown beyond counting; but, from the beginning, there has been a core of ministers and priests who shared the vision. Father Ed Kenny and Julia Pierson helped lay a solid foundation for the vision—and helped keep me going. They helped keep this Firesoul burning.

I'm sensitive to poverty and to the needs of the elderly because I was raised by my grandparents on Social Security and a pension for the blind. When I felt called to go into the ministry, my grandmother encouraged me, even though she was a widow by then and her blindness created special care needs. She said, "I know you can do it because God is with you." The neighbors said, "We'll watch your grandmother." And my older brother promised to care for our grandmother, so I was able to attend college and seminary. Members of my home church helped send me to college. People made significant sacrifices

Peace. Love. Serenity. Health. Safety. Contentment. Joy. Prosperity. All are mine as I walk the labyrinth. It simplifies life and allows solemn reflection. I am drawn back again and again.

Coming together is the beginning, keeping together is the process, working together is success.

for me to follow this path, and I've felt like my work to make life better for the elderly and poor is my way to show gratitude and pass it on. Not to mention that this is what churches should do. They should be socially active, and they should strive to change things for the better.

What has culminated as Stadium Place started nearly thirty years ago when I and a group of clergy in the Govans community all expressed the concern that some of our seniors had been abandoned by their families. Our elderly couldn't afford $100,000 entry fees to move into the expensive retirement communities that were sprouting up around us, and we thought, "We need to do something to help them." So we took an eyesore and turned it into Epiphany House, a home that could accommodate thirty seniors. The night we opened it, I sat in my car and watched far into the night because I was afraid someone might break in. Everything went fine, but we'd only been open two days when one of the seniors became ill, and we didn't have any place for her to go. Here the churches had provided this home and within just a couple of days, we were scratching around to find a nursing home.

We realized at that point that we still had a long way to go to be able to provide for all the needs the elderly have beyond just a place to live: health care, food, and spiritual sustenance. So we formed an organization called

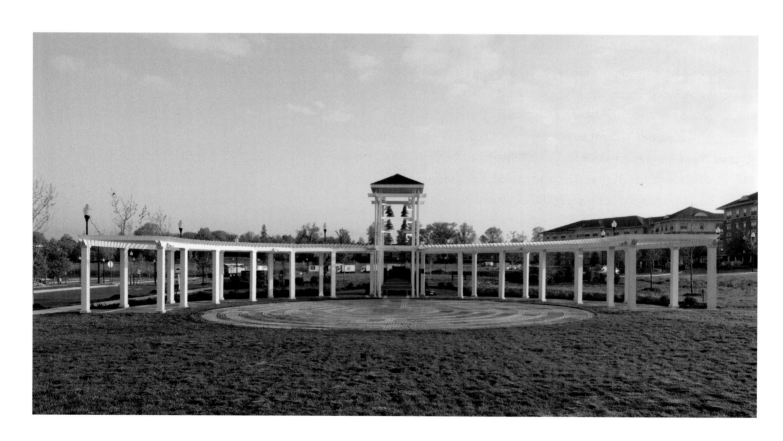

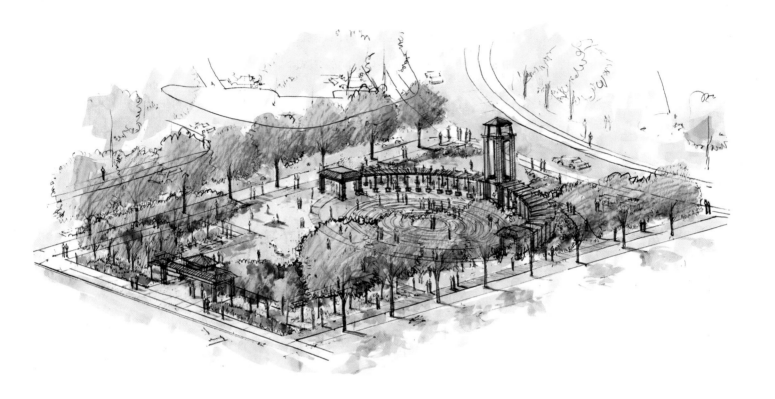

Govans Ecumenical Homes (GEH), consisting of seven Catholic and
Protestant churches. That organization grew into the Govans Ecumenical
Development Corporation (GEDCO), which now includes more than forty-five
congregations and community organizations, including synagogues. Over the
next years, GEDCO did a number of projects, including an emergency food
program and the creation of several more homes for the elderly, homeless, and
individuals with mental illness. These were all good projects, but we knew
that we had not yet achieved our goal of providing for the whole person—
body and soul—and our work convinced us that we needed more space
and economy of scale. So we prayed about it, as we went through a staff-led
strategic planning event.

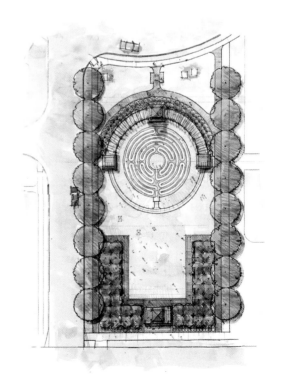

    Then the City of Baltimore put out a request for proposals to develop the
site of Memorial Stadium. This is where the Baltimore Orioles, Colts, and
Ravens had played for decades before the City built a new stadium; it had been
abandoned for about seven years. We knew right away that this thirty-three-
acre piece of land was exactly what we were looking for, so GEDCO entered
the competition. A tremendous amount of work went into the plan that we
presented to the City. It included going into the community to find out what

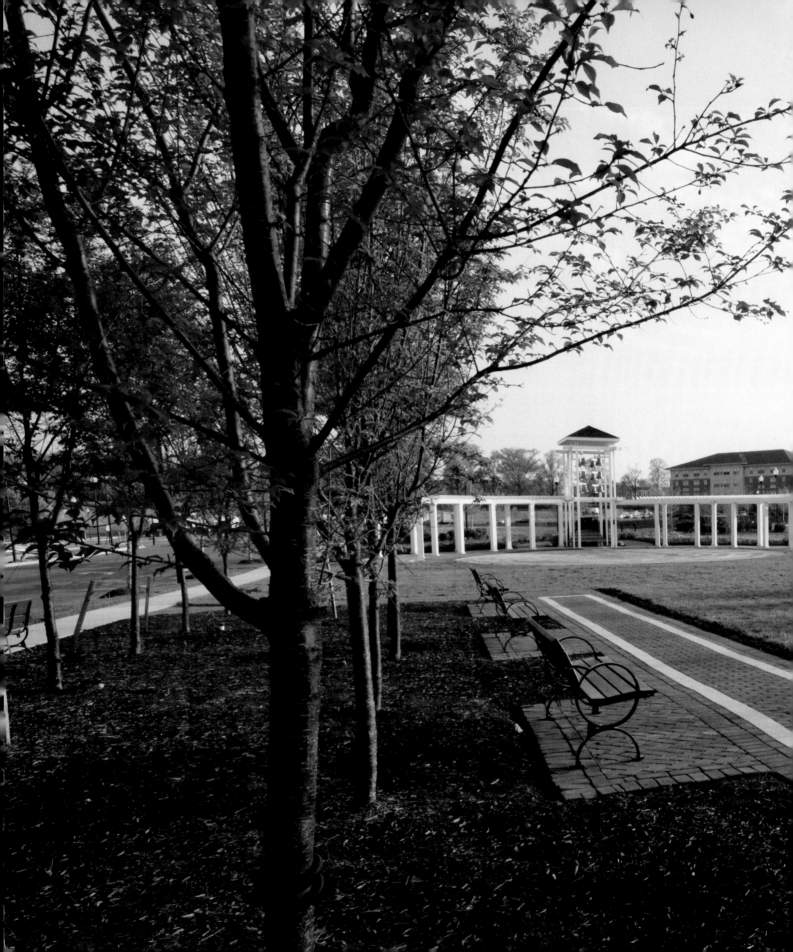

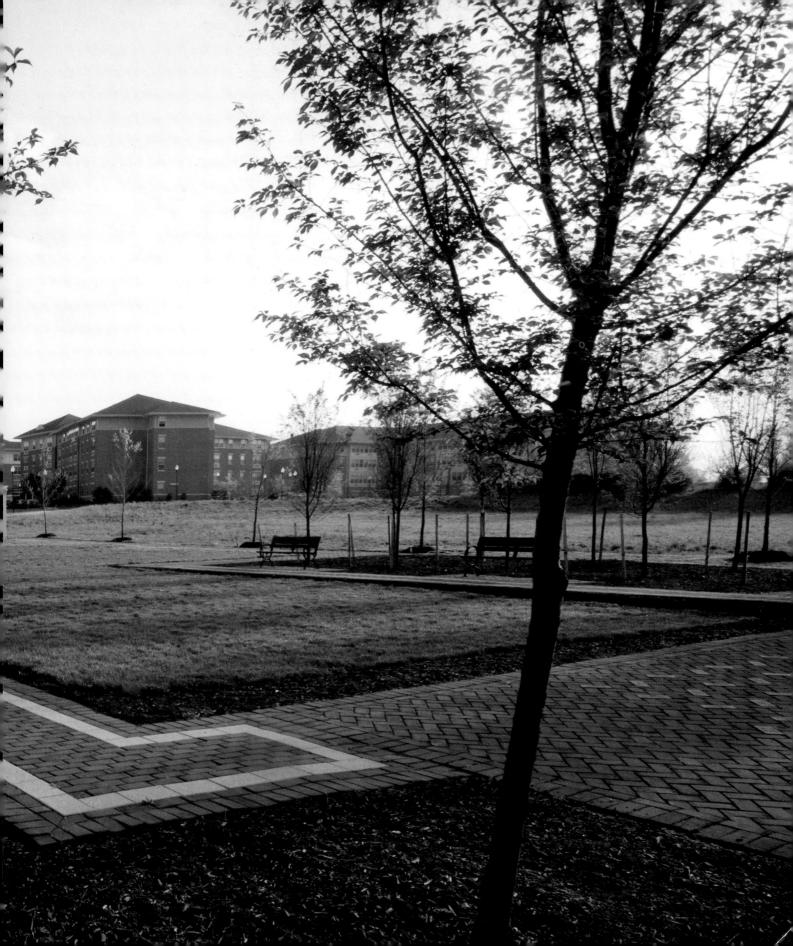

Father Creator and Mother Earth,
Thank you for your many blessings. I pray
for your continued guidance as I wander
on my journey . . . Help me to stay on the
path of enlightenment and to realize my full
potential in this earthly place of existence.

seniors would want as residents of this new housing complex. Almost every one of them asked if there would be a place for prayer and reflection, so the question of how to serve the spiritual side of people became a very important consideration in our planning.

It was at this point in the planning for Stadium Place—that's the name we gave to our vision for the senior housing complex—that I met Susan MacFarlane, who was serving with me on the Central Maryland Ecumenical Council. Susan is the kind of person who changes the feeling of a room when she walks into it. She can see God in every person and gives thanks for that. As a practitioner of Christian Science, Susan believes in the healing power of gratitude. She suggested that the spiritual center of this new development be ThanksGiving Place. There are two places dedicated to thanksgiving in the world, and Susan has visited both of them. One is located in Dallas, Texas. Known as the center of world thanksgiving, it is called Thanks-Giving Square. It is located on the exact center acre of the city and has gardens, fountains, and a large building that serves as a thanksgiving chapel. The second is the site of the Angel of Thanksgiving sculpture in Belfast, Ireland, a city long torn by the strife between Catholics and Protestants.

Susan thought that if we had a place dedicated to focusing on being grateful for all that we do have, it could only make our city better. Because gratitude reaches beyond any one religion, she thought that ThanksGiving Place would be perfect for the community we were planning. Not only is gratitude a core value for almost all people and all religions, it brings people together in a world where religion is often a divisive force. Studies have confirmed that when we're feeling grateful and we're expressing gratitude,

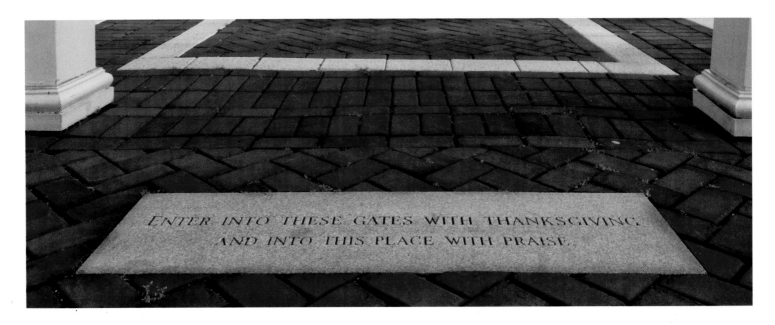

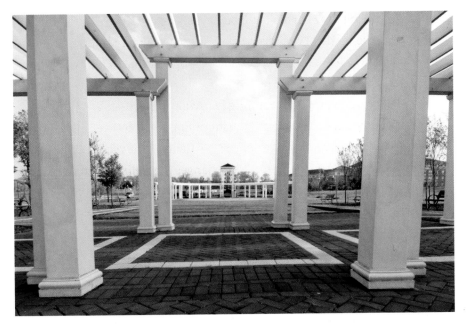

we're much healthier. The Stadium Place staff and board members liked the idea, so Susan and I created an interfaith committee to work on a design. The committee represented a wide range of faith groups, including individuals from various Christian faiths as well as from Jewish, Muslim, Buddhist, and Bahá'í communities. We held a charrette to get community input as well. Then we put all the ideas out on the table and started brainstorming.

Our first decision to make was "building or no building." It didn't take us long to figure out that having a structure meant heating, cooling, bathrooms, insurance, maintenance, and probably even the formation of a new corporation to keep it all running. We thought, "We could spend all our time raising money for a building, or we could come up with something much less costly and time-consuming that the seniors could help take care of and enjoy." So we voted for an outdoor space. We envisioned it not only serving the needs of residents, but also serving as a community resource. In all our planning research, the elderly in the neighborhood had made it clear that they wanted more safe places to walk: an outdoor space would provide that. Next we decided to have no religious symbols. Our first idea was to have plaques of all the known religions, but once we started to name them, we realized that we would undoubtedly leave one or more out. And how would we decide on the order? We just couldn't make that work, so no religions are named in ThanksGiving Place—making it a space open to all, with or without a religious belief.

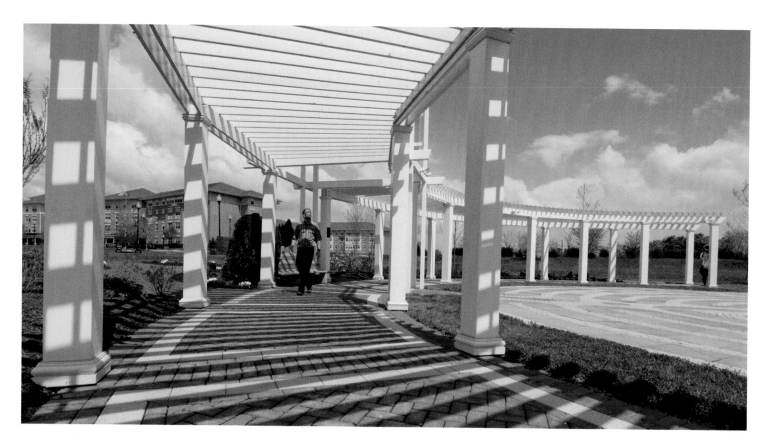

September 11, a year after our nation's great tragedy, and in my opinion stronger than ever, working side by side to beautify our land. Men and women, children of all ages and mental capacities. Different races and creeds and religions all together. Loving their country and most important of all, loving each other.

In the meantime, the battle for the right to develop Memorial Stadium was heating up. We had strong support from more than forty religious and neighborhood associations, and the YMCA became a vital component of our team. But we were pitted against some of the city's biggest developers. The night we made our presentation, more than six hundred people showed up to hear the presentations. As our presentation ended, the whole audience was waving their arms and singing "YMCA." We won—and what a victory that was! At that moment, two critically important things happened: TKF made a very generous grant for us to proceed with ThanksGiving Place, and the faith community came through marvelously with loans and grants.

Today, three buildings are up, and a fourth is under construction, providing rent-supported housing for 366 low-income seniors. More than two thousand people had applied to live at Stadium Place. In their applications, they hadn't written just their names; they had written who they were and why they wanted to live here. Some put praying hands on the cards and wrote things like, "Dear God, let me be chosen." For those who won the lottery, the move has been life-changing. Many of them have come from run-down, crime-infested areas of the city. In addition to housing, we offer doctor visits and serve nutritious meals. Those who want to buy groceries can take our shuttle bus to the supermarket. We have a computer center and a beauty shop. The

YMCA offers membership to our seniors at an incredibly low price, and they can go there for exercise, for classes, and for programs in the senior center.

At the spiritual heart of Stadium Place is ThanksGiving Place, a large square park that measures nearly an acre. As visitors enter, they pass a stone engraved with the words, "Enter this place with thanksgiving." Paths and gardens line both sides, benches are placed throughout, and covered areas and pergolas provide shade and shelter. Straight ahead, in the center, is our labyrinth. As soon as we made the decision to have an outdoor space, I thought of a labyrinth. We needed something neutral, and everyone on the committee could agree on a circle and a path as a metaphor for a journey, be it a faith journey or life's journey. A labyrinth can be used by a member of any faith or by a person with no faith. It can provide a place to relax, or it can be used on a spiritual quest for enlightenment. Many people can walk it at the same time, and it will mean something different to each one. The labyrinth at Thanks-Giving Place was designed to be flat, with the stones set into the ground, so that it is accessible for wheelchairs and seniors can walk it safely.

The seniors love to walk here or just sit and enjoy the beauty of the space. We have created a position for an intern to lead monthly labyrinth walks, and

Follow your path, your own path to enlightenment.

I was struck suddenly, as I was walking, with the reality that I sometimes feel I am walking in circles, when in fact, I am walking my own completely unique path. What a great metaphor for life.

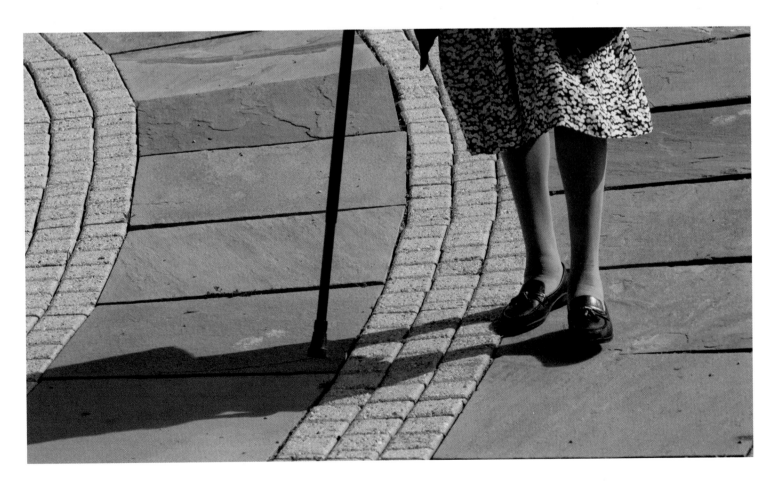

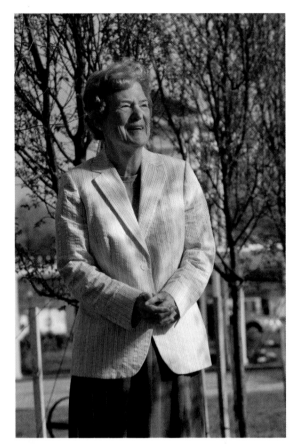

Susan MacFarlane, Firesoul

A quiet place where I can contemplate my future, learn to live with my pain, and plan for ways I can give back to others in these remaining years. Thank you for this place to reflect.

I will train some of the seniors so that they can show others how to use the labyrinth. People from the community are becoming more acquainted with it, and ThanksGiving Place is truly becoming the interfaith space we hoped it would be. All around the square are beautiful flower beds and trees. Now that the carillon has been installed, the bells literally call to all people to come to this place. Our plan is to have musicians play concerts during the warm months. We envision people coming from all over the city with chairs and blankets to sit on the lawn and listen—and perhaps give thanks.

Of all the wonderful ways that ThanksGiving Place can be used, one of the most important for both Susan MacFarlane and me is the event we have every year in November, at Thanksgiving time. As members of the Central Maryland Ecumenical Council, we were able to create an interfaith leadership award, to be presented at an interfaith breakfast at Stadium Place. The award is named in honor of two of the most prominent clergy persons of the last century in Baltimore: Cardinal Lawrence Shehan and Rabbi Jacob Agus, who were way ahead of their time in pushing for dialogue between Christians, Jews, and Muslims. On the Monday before Thanksgiving Day, we have a breakfast in one of the Stadium Place buildings; then everyone walks down to ThanksGiving Place for the presentation of the award. By magnifying the good in this way, we believe we're helping to create a better, more peaceful world.

And we're not done yet. We've just signed a contract with a developer to build 154 condominiums that we'll sell at below-market rates to seniors who want to live here for the rest of their lives and take part in the community of Stadium Place. We also plan to create some affinity commercial space next to ThanksGiving Place—space for a dentist, a podiatrist, a chiropractor, and, God willing, an assisted or skilled living home for people who can't be cared for in their rooms. The model we hope to use is called a "Green House," an innovative and non-institutional design that truly enhances the quality of life for the elders. Finally, we plan to have a restaurant/café overlooking the labyrinth and gardens, which we hope will attract more people to this space and fulfill our vision of it as an interfaith and community gathering place.

One of my earliest personal memories is of being on a tricycle—just a tiny child sitting on a tiny tricycle on Third Street in Wilmington, Delaware. And my grandfather is sitting on the porch of his house watching me. Over the years, it has dawned on me that my grandfather wasn't alone in that memory. There were old men and women sitting on porches and steps all up and down the street, watching children play.

Not long ago, on a spring evening, I attended a meeting at Stadium Place. When the meeting ended and I walked out of the building, the sun was setting in the west. On the porches there were old men and women, sitting and watching children play—the YMCA soccer teams on the field and the neighborhood children on the playground, the playground that more than two thousand people in the community had helped build. And down the hill, ThanksGiving Place glittered like gold in the setting sun. I had stepped back into my childhood memory, and I thought, "This is it. It took us thirty years to get here, but this is what we wanted."

Maybe this is the culmination of my ministry—but it isn't the end. Who knows what life has in store for us? What I do know is that my ministry won't stop until I die. It's what I like doing, and I think it keeps me healthy. Certainly, it keeps me happy.

I leave feeling more peaceful, refreshed, better than when I arrived. How thankful I am.

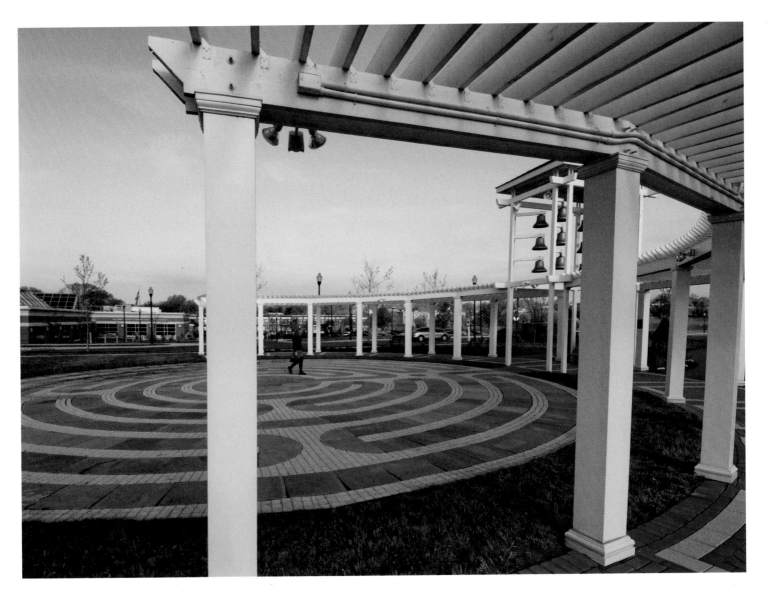

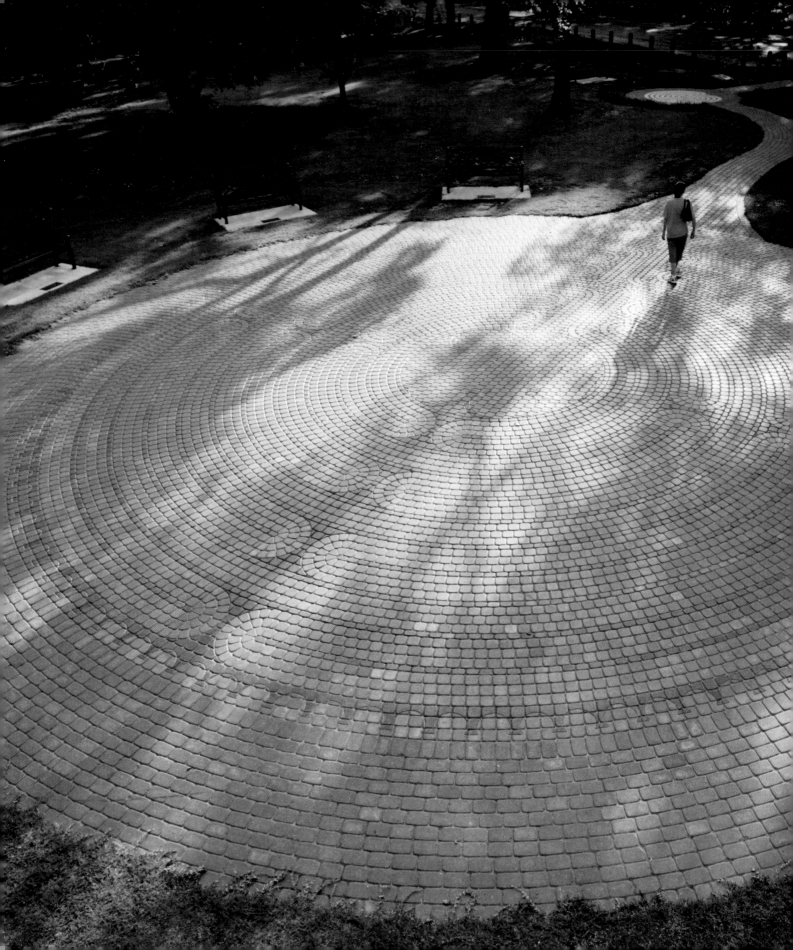